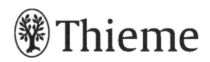

Noninterpretive Skills in Radiology

Q&A Top Score Prep Guide for the Boards

Alan F. Weissman, MD
Desert Radiology
Las Vegas, Nevada

Twyla B. Bartel, DO, MBA, FACNM
Global Advanced Imaging, PLLC
Little Rock, Arkansas

42 illustrations

Thieme
New York • Stuttgart• Delhi • Rio de Janeiro

Executive Editor: William Lamsback
Managing Editor: J. Owen Zurhellen IV
Associate Managing Editor: Kenneth Schubach
Director, Editorial Services: Mary Jo Casey
Production Editor: Torsten Scheihagen
International Production Director: Andreas Schabert
Vice President, Editorial and E-Product
      Development: Vera Spillner
International Marketing Director: Fiona Henderson
International Sales Director: Louisa Turrell
Director of Sales, North America: Mike Roseman
Senior Vice President and Chief Operating
      Officer: Sarah Vanderbilt
President: Brian D. Scanlan
Illustrator: Twyla B. Bartel
Printer: Everbest Printing Co.

Library of Congress Cataloging-in-Publication Data

Names: Weissman, Alan, MD, author. | Bartel, Twyla B., author.
Title: Noninterpretive skills in radiology : Q & A top score prep guide
      for the boards / Alan Weissman, Twyla B. Bartel.
Description: New York : Thieme, [2016] | Includes bibliographical
      references and index.
Identifiers: LCCN 2016035755 (print) | LCCN 2016037357 (ebook)
      | ISBN 9781626234598 (pbk.) | ISBN 9781626234604 (eISBN) |
      ISBN 9781626234604 (E-book)
Subjects: | MESH: Radiology | Clinical Competence | Examination
      Questions
Classification: LCC RC78.15 (print) | LCC RC78.15 (ebook) | NLM WN
      18.2 | DDC 616.07/57076--dc23
LC record available at https://lccn.loc.gov/2016035755

Thieme Publishers New York
333 Seventh Avenue, New York, NY 10001 USA
+1 800 782 3488, customerservice@thieme.com

Thieme Publishers Stuttgart
Rüdigerstrasse 14, 70469 Stuttgart, Germany
+49 [0]711 8931 421, customerservice@thieme.de

Thieme Publishers Delhi
A-12, Second Floor, Sector-2, Noida-201301
Uttar Pradesh, India
+91 120 45 566 00, customerservice@thieme.in

Thieme Publishers Rio de Janeiro, Thieme Publicações Ltda.
Edifício Rodolpho de Paoli, 25º andar
Av. Nilo Peçanha, 50 – Sala 2508
Rio de Janeiro 20020-906 Brasil
+55 21 3172-2297 / +55 21 3172-1896

Cover design: Thieme Publishing Group
Typesetting by DiTech Process Solutions

Printed in China by Everbest Printing Co.   5 4 3 2 1

ISBN 978-1-62623-459-8

Also available as an e-book:
eISBN 978-1-62623-460-4

Important note: Medicine is an ever-changing science undergoing continual development. Research and clinical experience are continually expanding our knowledge, in particular our knowledge of proper treatment and drug therapy. Insofar as this book mentions any dosage or application, readers may rest assured that the authors, editors, and publishers have made every effort to ensure that such references are in accordance with **the state of knowledge at the time of production of the book**.

Nevertheless, this does not involve, imply, or express any guarantee or responsibility on the part of the publishers in respect to any dosage instructions and forms of applications stated in the book. **Every user is requested to examine carefully** the manufacturers' leaflets accompanying each drug and to check, if necessary in consultation with a physician or specialist, whether the dosage schedules mentioned therein or the contraindications stated by the manufacturers differ from the statements made in the present book. Such examination is particularly important with drugs that are either rarely used or have been newly released on the market. Every dosage schedule or every form of application used is entirely at the user's own risk and responsibility. The authors and publishers request every user to report to the publishers any discrepancies or inaccuracies noticed. If errors in this work are found after publication, errata will be posted at www.thieme.com on the product description page.

Some of the product names, patents, and registered designs referred to in this book are in fact registered trademarks or proprietary names even though specific reference to this fact is not always made in the text. Therefore, the appearance of a name without designation as proprietary is not to be construed as a representation by the publisher that it is in the public domain.

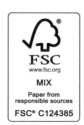

Contents

Preface

The radiology boards are tough. With the already staggering information mountain each of us must climb to pass the traditional boards, why would the American Board of Radiology (ABR) pile on yet another new section—in fact, a section in which most radiologists have little formal training?

Because the ABR knows exactly what it is doing.

The Non-Interpretive Skills (NIS) section is the latest addition to the ABR boards, and the NIS is important stuff. Seasoned radiologists on the front lines can attest that there is a lot more to thriving in a successful radiology practice than just "reading 'em right." There are quality issues, safety issues, and HIPAA compliance issues. There are contrast reactions, MRI contraindications, and legal matters. There are interactions with your patients and staff, informatics, and professionalism.

And if you haven't yet come to the realization that a business background is a big advantage in the world of practicing medicine, you will. Healthcare represents 17% of the gross national product, and everyone wants a piece. To compete, we must see that with medicine, there is a product, a customer, an opportunity for efficiency, and a chance to develop value. For the NIS, we are not tasked with studying the macroeconomics of medicine, but we are required to understand the language of the statistics, the metrics, and the jargon used to continually improve our systems.

These issues have been smoldering for years. The medical establishment has finally mandated knowledge of this material, and, fortunately, the ABR does a great job of defining the requirements.

The topics covered here are taken directly from the ABR syllabus. We examine the topics and explain the key points of what you need to know.

We also take our best shot at keeping all of you engaged (through plain speak and real radiology examples), so that learning the NIS is sort of fun. (Can we at least agree on "not too painful"?) The first half of the book discusses select principles in text format. The second half of the book reinforces concepts and adds more, through a Question and Answer format. Memory aids in the form of mnemonics and tips are scattered throughout. If you are the type that likes them, that's great. If not, then brush them aside, stick to the facts, and you will be fine.

The ABR points out that this material is an ever-changing target. It would be a daunting task to attempt a Six Sigma goal of interactive educational immersion with this book (you will read about Six Sigma on page 5), but let's say we set our goal at three standard deviations (SDs), or within 99.7%, of the required educational material.

At the most recent Radiological Society of North America (RSNA), I attended an interesting lecture concerning the new NIS, given by several board examiners. The boards' aims are not at all punitive, and there is no quota for required "fails." The board strives for thoughtful licensing of those radiologists who demonstrate both competence and safety. This honorable goal ultimately protects society. By this book's end, we are confident that you will feel prepared to pass the NIS portion of the exam, and as an equally important goal, we hope that you take with you to your practice a better understanding of that special skill set in radiology "beyond the diagnosis." Happy reading!

Alan F. Weissman, MD

Twyla B. Bartel, MD

1 Introduction to Noninterpretive Skills

Quality: It's All about Quality Improvement

The NIS primarily concerns itself with core quality and safety.

Quality control (QC), quality assurance (QA), and quality improvement (QI) sound kind of similar, but they are not the same thing. The most up-to-date process is QI. This is the only one of the three that results in an improved system.

Tip: Remember that QI is the current and best iteration because it is the only one with "improvement" in the title.

Quality Control

QC defines the acceptable parameters. For example, the QC of a lumbar puncture includes that "sterile technique must be strictly followed." The QC won't tell you the best way to confirm sterile technique, and if infection does occur, the QC won't give blame or provide fixes. The QC is simply "the rules."

Quality Assurance

QA is better than QC (although still not as progressive as QI) and is a method of monitoring feedback. For example, telling one of your residents, "Peter, you overcall cardiomegaly on chest X-rays all the time," is a form of (fairly blunt) quality assurance. Peter may take some solace in knowing that your comment nicely exemplifies key points of QA: reactive, usually retrospective, involves policing (and sometimes punishing) and determines who is at fault. QA is a stable process and, by itself, doesn't necessarily bring about change.

Quality Improvement

QI is a method to actually change the problematic process. For example, telling Peter the resident, "For the next 10 chest X-ray cases, you need to measure and confirm an enlarged cardiothoracic ratio before concluding that the heart is enlarged," is a simple form of QI. This method is the best, since it results in change. QI is both retrospective and prospective, avoids attributing blame, creates systems that prevent errors from happening, and is a more recent phenomenon in healthcare.[2]

A Few Organizations and a Few Acronyms

The Institute of Medicine (IOM) is a nonprofit organization that provides independent and objective analysis and advice to inform public policy decisions related to science, technology, and medicine.[3] The IOM has defined six quality aims for medical care, and you have to know this list.

The six quality aims of the IOM are as follows:

1. Safe
2. Timely
3. Equitable
4. Effective
5. Efficient
6. Patient centered

The acronym STEEEP is provided by the institute to remember these quality aims.

Tip: If you find it tough to remember what this acronym stands for, especially with three nonspecific "Es" in a row, try this mnemonic (**Fig. 1.1**).

The Accreditation Council for Graduate Medical Education (ACGME) and the 24 American Board of Medical Specialties (ABMS) agree that a physician must demonstrate the following six core competencies for Graduate Medical Education (GME) and Maintenance of Certification (MOC). Here is the second list you must know.[4] (In fact, all board-certified physicians in the United States must know this list.)

The six core competencies of MOC are:

1. Patient care
2. Medical knowledge
3. Interpersonal and communication skills
4. Professionalism
5. Systems-based practice
6. Practice-based learning and improvement

The ABMS provides the mnemonic "Knowledge CLiPS."

Tip: Try this alternative mnemonic (**Fig. 1.2**).

Adopted from the ABMS website, here is a little more elaboration on these core competencies.

1. *Patient care:* Provide compassionate, appropriate, and effective treatment.

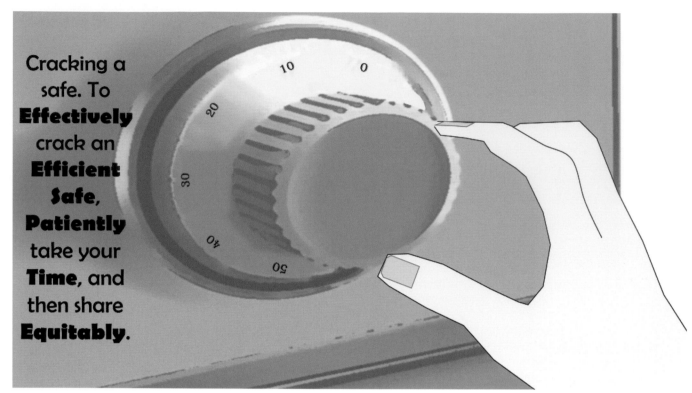

Fig. 1.1 Mnemonic device for the six quality aims of the IOM. Effective, efficient, safe, patient-centered, timely, and equitable.

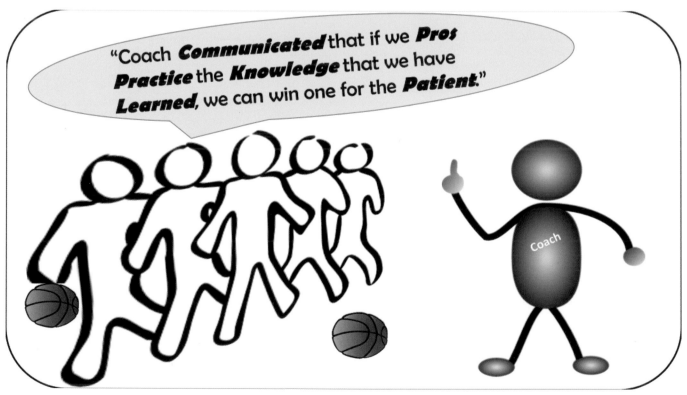

Fig. 1.2 Mnemonic device for the six core competencies of MOC. Communication, professionalism, practice (systems-based), knowledge, learning (practice-based), and patient-care.

2. *Medical knowledge:* Demonstrate knowledge about established and evolving healthcare science.
3. *Interpersonal and communication skills:* Demonstrate skills that result in effective information exchange with patients, families, and professional associates, and use effective listening skills to work as both a team member and at times a leader.
4. *Professionalism:* Demonstrate a commitment to carry out professional responsibility, ethics, and sensitivity to diverse populations.
5. *Systems based practice:* Demonstrate awareness of the larger context and systems of healthcare, and optimally utilize those systems to improve care.
6. *Practice-based learning and improvement:* Demonstrate the ability to investigate and evaluate patient care practices, assess scientific evidence, and improve the practice of medicine.

Business Intelligence

The common denominator for these required terms is business intelligence.

Best Practices

Best practice is a method that consistently shows results superior to those achieved with other means, and that method is used as a benchmark.[5] "Best practice" has recently become something of a buzzword in business. Best practice examples for employee satisfaction might include creating a culture of engagement, promoting health and well-being, and reducing employee stress.

Tip: A best practice continually evolves.

Dashboards

Dashboards are visual displays of the most important information consolidated into a single screen.[6] We might think of this as radiology specific (for example, radiology case list, relative value units [RVUs] completed today, and permitted turnaround time per study), but dashboards have much broader utility for any business. A good dashboard can save a company time and money, if the dashboard is exactly tailored to the required industry specs.

Tip: All quality dashboards have immediacy, intuitiveness, and simplicity.

Benchmarking

Benchmarking is the measurement of the quality of an organization's policies and strategies and their comparison with standard measurements. One goal of a benchmark is to determine where improvements are needed. Another goal is to analyze how other organizations achieve their success.[7]

Tip: In radiology, turnaround time, critical findings compliance, and peer review expectations are examples of benchmarks.

Value

Driven by economics, "value" has grown into a popular medical industry term.[8] As it relates to healthcare, value is defined as the following:

Value = (service □ quality)/cost.

A good value from a patient's perspective might include interacting with polite radiology staff and receiving quality image interpretation at a reasonable price.

Radiology example

Cash-pay whole-body screening MRI is probably *not* a good value. The yield is generally low and the cost is generally high.

Real-life example

A $200,000+ European sports car may be of very high quality, but purchasing one is probably not a good value. Top-notch cars like these generally have a low "benefits-to-cost" ratio. Put another way: value = outcomes/cost. For our purposes in radiology, value is directly proportional to optimal appropriateness, good outcomes, improved efficiency, and cost reduction.

It is worth noting that the formerly voluntary physician quality reporting system (PQRS) is now an actual metric used to determine pay.

Tip: Centers for Medicare & Medicaid Services (CMS) is starting to pay for value rather than simply for volume.

Key Performance Indicators

Key performance indicators (KPIs) are business metrics used to evaluate factors that are vital to the success of an organization.[9] These include both financial and nonfinancial measures integral to defining an organization's mission and strategy.

KPIs help us measure how well companies, business units, projects, and individuals are performing compared to their strategic goals and objectives. Well-designed KPIs provide the vital navigation instruments that clearly demonstrate current levels of performance.

Radiology example

KPIs might include customer satisfaction, average call wait time, and call abandonment.

Tip: You can't manage what you can't measure.

Business Intelligence in Practice

Your office manager informs you that customers complain about their MRI experiences. She says that patients feel like they aren't getting a good *value*. They like the quality of the reads, but think the staff are rude, scheduling takes too long, and the co-pays are too high. These are some of the *KPIs*.

Fortunately, your manager is immediately aware of all patient issues, since her computer is equipped with a *dashboard* to easily view daily patient comments, days out for scheduling, and daily co-pays.

Addressing one of these three issues, she tells you that the regional *benchmark* for getting a patient scanned (from the time the patient makes the call until the actual scan takes place) is 3 days. Since your office is currently operating at 4 days out, she sets "2 days or better" as her goal.

Her bigger picture aim is to have the most satisfied radiology customer base in the region. Improving the three KPIs listed above will help bring her closer to achieving a *best practice* office for others to emulate.

Useful Approaches to Quality Improvement

A successful program must have the entire organization commit to QI. Although this begins with leadership, good leaders know that involvement of frontline workers in the solutions is key, because no one understands the problems like they do.

As physicians, we are all very familiar with the scientific method and how it leads to logical conclusions. Variations of this theme are used in business and organizational operations.

Plan, Do, Study, Act (PDSA) Cycle

This is the standard cycle for testing changes in QI (and is basically the scientific method). Plan the test or objective, do the test, study the results, and then act (either adopt the change, modify, and try again, or abandon the change). The PDSA cycle, also known as the improvement cycle, is a powerful tool for learning.[10]

Tip: The ABR advocates using the PDSA cycle for their practice QI (PQI) projects.

You can use PDSA cycles to test an idea by temporarily invoking a change and assessing its impact.

Example: Your patients complain that the information sheet you require them to fill out is too long. You then review the sheet and identify possible unnecessary questions (Plan). Then, you make some modifications to shorten the sheet (Do). Then, you test the new sheet out on a small number of patients. You also make sure that you and the other interpreting radiologists are still satisfied (Study). Then, if the new sheets are satisfactory, you incorporate them into a larger segment of the practice. Finally, if the results of the larger study remain satisfactory, you implement the new sheets practice-wide (Act).

Tip: Start small with the PDSA cycle. Initially, use a limited sample population to make sure your solution works. In the long run, this saves time, money, and risk.

Lean

Lean is the "relentless elimination of waste." Lean can also be thought of as a method of "making obvious what adds value by reducing everything else." The Lean principles of process improvement were first described in the manufacturing industry with Toyota automobiles, but translate very well into operations in general. Lean focuses on a smooth workflow and relies on engaging the whole workforce.[11] This technique lends itself nicely to radiology, where many people work as a team to produce the final product. Core principles of Lean include eliminating waste, engaging and simplifying, and respecting all people (i.e., customers, employees, and suppliers).

Tip: With Lean, if you respect all people, then you don't need to remember the "important ones."

Some specific elements of Lean are discussed below.

"Pull"

This means do the work only when the next step is ready. There should be no work in progress inventory.

Example: Reading a follow-up positron emission tomography/computed tomography (PET/CT) scan without comparison on a patient after his third round of chemotherapy is not optimal. Clearly, there is a comparison around somewhere. Here, the next step is not ready and the comparison should have already been obtained.

"Just in time"

This means to deliver materials only when needed.

Example: Most radiology departments staff the number of radiologists per shift based on historic and usually predictable study volumes. If your CT tech instead batches 15 trauma CT scans, this creates both turnaround time and physician stress problems. Here, the CT tech batched studies rather than delivering them on a regular schedule.

"Kanban"

Kanban means maintaining inventory levels. Processes must have a signal to indicate when supplies need replenishing.

Example: You are scrubbed in the middle of a lumbar puncture on an obese patient and suddenly decide that you need a longer spinal needle. But when you ask for one, the tech explains that there aren't any and that someone probably used the last one. Here, this preventable problem needed a "Kanban" mechanism to signal low supply.

"Standard work"

This means to reduce unnecessary variation.

Example: If every office in your practice has its own separate policies, then rotating techs and radiologists will probably need more time to acclimate, become more frustrated, and even make more errors. By the way, the suggestion to minimize variation is concordant with current American College of Radiology (ACR) directives. Standardized reporting throughout the country is now gaining momentum.

Six Sigma

Six Sigma is another highly regarded improvement methodology. This was first used at Motorola and then perfected under CEO Jack Welsh at General Electric.

Sigma is the Greek letter often used in statistics and refers to the normal distribution of mathematical outcomes.[13]

"Six Sigma" targets an extremely low defect rate of 3.4 per million opportunities, which represents six standard deviations (SDs) from the population average. In percentages, this means that 99.99966% of the work is done correctly.

As a reminder, one SD equals 68%, two SDs equal 95%, and three SDs equal 99.7% of the data.

Six Sigma is an extremely lofty goal. The real point is to strive for near perfection.

Tip: Like all QI, Six Sigma work is never completed, because a system is never truly "perfected."

Define, Measure, Analyze, Improve, and Control (DMAIC) Methodology

This data-driven quality strategy is an integral part of Six Sigma, but can also be a stand-alone process.[14]

Tip: Lean and Six Sigma share similar methodologies and tools, but there are differences. Lean management is focused on eliminating waste, while Six Sigma management is focused on eliminating defects.

The Eight Wastes in Lean

The standard acronym for these wastes is TIM WOODS.[12]

Value Added or Non–Value Added

Every activity conducted in a business is either value added (VA) or non–value added (NVA). VA activities are those that physically transform a product or service in the eyes of a customer. NVA activities are those that do not. Although some of these may be essential "behind the scenes" activities, they are still considered NVA and encompass waste. The following section discusses examples of NVA activities (waste).

Transport

Movement of product should be controlled by time and distance.

Example: Waiting for hospital transport to bring the patient to radiology is often the rate-limiting step.

Another example: Placing an ultrasound room physically distant from the radiology reading room wastes both sonographer and patient time.

Inventory

Producing inventory that does not immediately move to the next process is NVA.

Example: An interventional radiology department with inaccurate supply need estimations will waste money on expired products.

Motion

Excessive movement of operator and equipment is waste.

Example: A suboptimal computer interface requiring extra clicks to load your cases is NVA.

Another example: Driving a portable X-ray machine to patients' homes may be prohibitively slow.

Waiting

Waiting should be minimized.

Example: Your system requires the ultrasound tech to enter information on a shared computer after the scan, but before presenting the case to the radiologist. The ultrasound tech may need to wait until that computer is free, and this NVA activity costs the company money.

Overproduction

Product should not exceed demand.

Example: Opening up a new but poorly conceived office that results in few referrals and scans is an example of overproduction.

Overprocessing

This waste results from poor tool or product design. If you don't know what your customer wants, how can you possibly create the most desired product?

Example: The referring foot and ankle orthopedic surgeon *only* wants a "limited bone scan of the feet and ankles." He specifically does not want a standard whole-body bone scan (because he doesn't want to deal with the incidental findings often picked up on a whole-body scan). Performing the standard whole-body scan on his patients takes extra time and upsets your customer.

Defects

Errors are waste. It usually takes less time to get it right the first time than it does to correct the errors.

Example: Making a sloppy error in a dictation as the result of a hurried effort may require dealing with time-consuming, irate phone calls from referring physicians and ultimately lead to a loss of confidence and business from referring services.

Skills

Failure to optimize skill sets with work duties is non-value added (NVA).

Example: As a physician, using your time to look up and dial referring service offices is NVA. Use an assistant, and stick to the highest and best use of your training.

Another example: Delegating tasks to the unqualified is also NVA. Using low-paid, poorly trained employees to handle interactive patient scheduling (which is often quite complex) is usually not worth the trade-off between perceived "cost savings" and resultant unhappy customers.

Seven Tools of Quality Improvement

There are *seven* basic tools of QI. These are a fixed set of graphical techniques identified as the most helpful to troubleshoot issues related to quality. These are termed "basic" because they are intended for people with little formal training to find useful.[15]

Before discussing the seven methodologies of QI, let's first examine "the five whys." Most problems have more than one cause and, to really solve the problem, you need to find that underlying cause. You can often identify the source of the problem using the five whys. This begins with the initial question of why something bad happened. This continues with follow-up why questions.

"The Five Whys" in Action

Example: A STAT CT head wasn't read within the contractually promised 1 hour, and the emergency room (ER) department complains. The simple move is to blame the radiologist on duty, or conclude that the radiology department is understaffed at that time. But maybe there is more to the story.

You ask the radiologist, "Why didn't you read it?" He responds, "Because the study was incomplete and was missing images."

You then ask the tech, "Why was the study incomplete?"

The tech at the hospital responds, "Well, I sent it, but I have no way of knowing if all of the images crossed over."

You then ask the supervising tech, "Why doesn't the tech have any way of knowing if all of the images crossed over?" The supervising tech responds, "There actually is a way to tell. The tech working tonight is a rotating tech and must not know how to find that information." Mystery solved. (Here, only three "whys" were needed to get to the root of the problem.)

The supervisor then trains the tech on duty and develops a training plan for subsequent rotating techs.

The seven tools of QI are as follows:

1. Flow chart
2. Cause-and-effect diagram

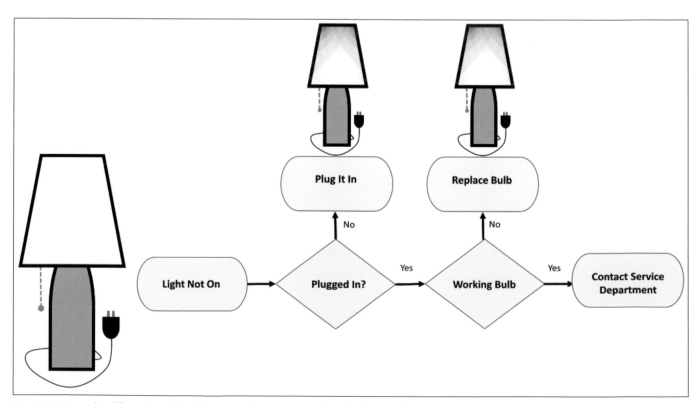

Fig. 1.3 Example of flowchart. Algorithm depicts steps needed to fix a light bulb.

3. Check sheet
4. Control chart
5. Histogram
6. Pareto chart
7. Scatter diagram

Tip: Most quality issues can be solved with these seven basic tools of QI.

1. *Flow chart:* This is the typical algorithm, and is a picture of the separate steps of a process in sequential order (**Fig. 1.3**).
2. *Cause-and-effect diagram:* This is also known as a fishbone or Ishikawa diagram. (Dr. Ishikawa was a professor of engineering at Tokyo University and a pioneer in QI.) The fishbone diagram identifies many possible causes for a problem, helps to structure a brainstorming session, and immediately sorts ideas into useful categories. The five whys are often invoked in a fishbone diagram (**Fig. 1.4**).
3. *Check sheet:* This is a structured, prepared form for collecting and analyzing data (**Fig. 1.5**).
4. *Control chart:* This is a graph used to study how a process changes over time. The data are plotted in chronological order. Using historical data, a control chart has a central line to illustrate deviations from the average, an upper line for the upper control limit, and a lower line for the lower control limit. This differentiates common causes of variation from special causes for variation (**Fig. 1.6**).
5. *Histogram:* This is the most commonly used graph to show frequency distributions in the context of two variables. This represents the distribution by mean. If the histogram is normal, the graph takes the shape of a bell curve. Any variation from the bell curve is abnormal, and may take an array of shapes, such as right-sided skewed, bimodal, or even dog-food shaped (**Fig. 1.7**).
6. *Pareto diagram:* A Pareto diagram is a bar graph. The lengths of the bars represent the frequency or cost (i.e., time or money) of each variable and are arranged with the longest bars on the left and the shortest bars on the right. This graph visually depicts which situations are most significant, permitting appropriate channeling of resources to fix the problem (**Fig. 1.8**).
7. *Scatter diagram:* A scatter diagram graphs pairs of numerical data, with one variable on each axis, to

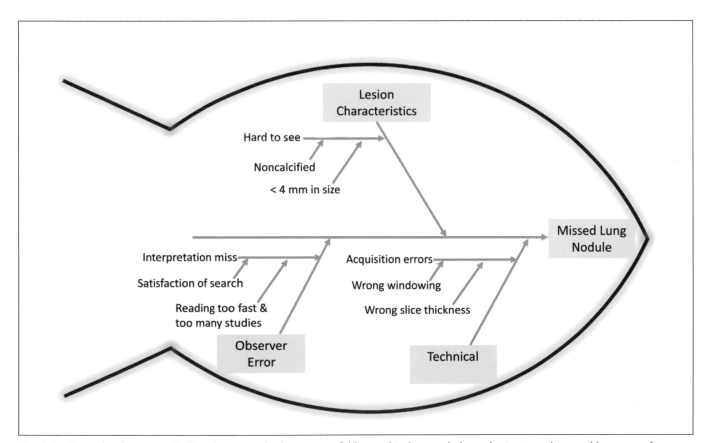

Fig. 1.4 Example of cause-and-effect diagram. Also known as a fishbone, this diagram helps to brainstorm the possible causes of a missed lung nodule.

Interventional Radiology Procedure Delays

REASONS	Monday	Tuesday	Wednesday	Thursday	Friday
Busy Time of Day	I	IIII	I		II
Technical Problems	II	III		IIII	II
Untrained Staff	IIII		IIII	II	
TOTALS	7	8	6	7	4

Fig. 1.5 Example of check sheet. This structured form assists in collecting and analyzing data to explain interventional radiology delays.

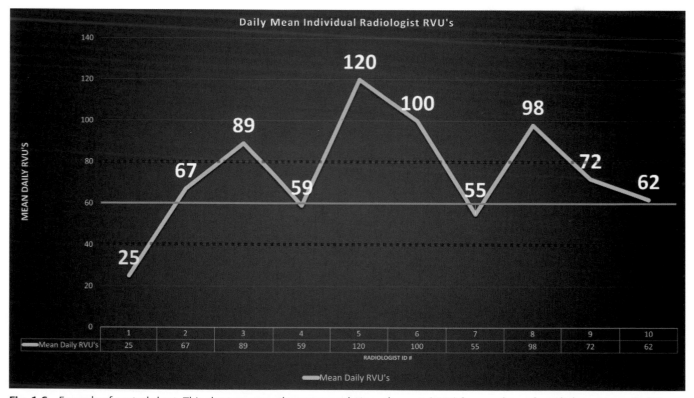

Fig. 1.6 Example of control chart. This chart assesses the average relative value unit (RVU) for members of a radiology group. Radiologist 1 falls below the normal control limit.

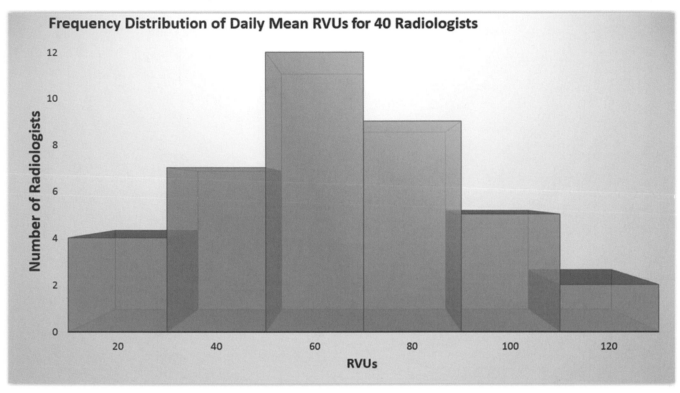

Fig. 1.7 Example of histogram. The graph shows the distribution of daily mean RVUs for 40 radiologists.

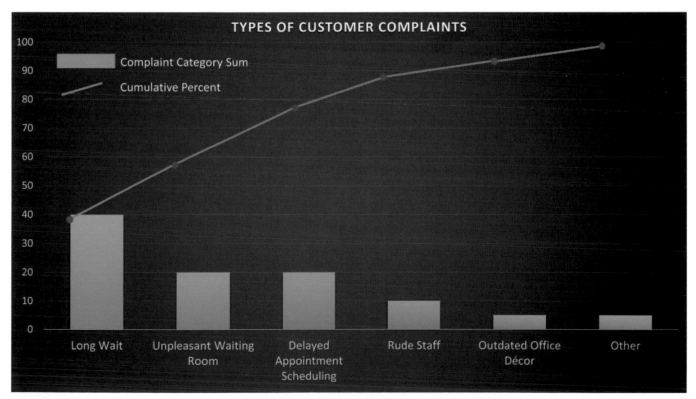

Fig. 1.8 Example of Pareto diagram. This graphically depicts the most significant causes of customer complaints. *Types of customer complaints*: Long wait (40%), unpleasant waiting room, delayed appointment scheduling, rude staff, outdated office décor, other. In this example, customer complaints could be decreased by 80% if only the first three problems are addressed.

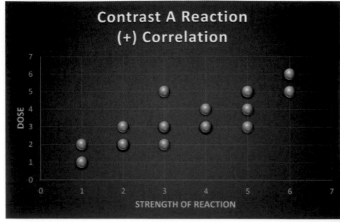

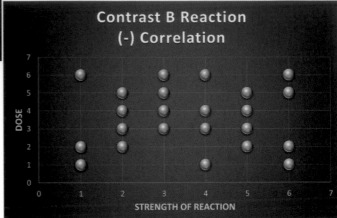

Fig. 1.9 Example of scatter diagrams. They demonstrate a good correlation between the dose of contrast A and reactions, but a poor correlation between the dose of contrast B and reactions.

look for a relationship between them. This can be useful when trying to identify potential root causes of problems (**Fig. 1.9**).

Safety

The Joint Commission (TJC; formerly JACHO) issues national safety goals in medicine. There are a lot of important boards, but this one is really important, because if your institution is not TJC accredited, you lose funding and cannot run your business.

TJC is independent, not for profit, and accredits 21,000 healthcare facilities in the United States. Its vision statement is, "All people always experience the safest, highest quality, best value healthcare across all settings."

In general terms, one of the bigger building blocks of the NIS is safety. Although safety concerns certainly didn't originate in 1998, that year a landmark article was published (by the Institute of Medicine [IOM]), which revealed a shocking number of deaths resulting from medical-related errors. This article, entitled, "To err is human: building a safer health system," brought about many positive changes in healthcare.[17]

The article had two key points. First, many deaths per year (44,000–98,000) were attributable to medical errors. For perspective, more people die in a given year as a result of medical errors than from either motor vehicle accidents (43,000) or breast cancer (42,000).

Second, the cause of these errors usually wasn't bad people working in good healthcare systems, but rather, good people working in bad healthcare systems.

Tip: Most errors are preventable with operational changes.

Safety versus Error

Safety and error are a little bit different. *Safety* is defined as "freedom from accidental injury." *Error* is defined as "failure of a planned action to be completed as intended," or "use of the wrong plan to achieve an aim."

The Hidden Troubles with Errors

In addition to potentially harming the patient, errors cost money and injure the public's trust in the system.

On a more personal level, errors can cause you (as the radiologist) real problems.

Example: Say that you missed a cancer on a CT scan, and that your miss really did lead to the patient's death. You will probably feel awful. Harboring shame and guilt, you might try to keep it a secret from friends and colleagues, and that adds stress. Plus, there is a decent chance that you will get sued. You are now the "*second victim*." Healthcare professionals pay for their mistakes, in part, with psychological discomfort. This is similar to posttraumatic stress disorder, and this type of guilt and stress has been known to cause significant morbidity, including suicide. In these cases, it is important for others who are aware of the situation to console.[18]

Four Fundamental Factors Leading to Errors

The IOM article concluded that four fundamental factors typically led to errors. The mnemonic *SLLaP* was provided for these factors, and this stands for system, licensing, liability, and payment.

Tip: You can also remember SLLaP, as in getting slapped across the face for making an error (**Fig. 1.10**).

System

This refers to the lack of a single system. Medicine is unfortunately often fragmented, or a "nonsystem."

For example, when a patient shops from doctor to doctor, loss of information is commonplace. Non-system loss of information may also result from causes beyond the patient's control (e.g., a change in the company insurance plan).

Licensing

Licensing exams have historically neglected to actually focus on medical errors. This problem is currently being rectified (as evidenced by our own NIS exam).

Liability

Legal issues frighten us into concealing our mistakes, so as a group, we usually lose the opportunity to learn from our colleague's errors.

Payment

This refers to the failure of third-party payers to provide incentives (i.e., financial rewards) for safety.

Safe move: Organizations often name a "safety champion." That individual is responsible for owning the safety processes and overseeing the safety reporting system.

Errors

Adverse Event

This is an injury caused by medical care and does not necessarily imply error or blame.

Examples: Pneumothorax post thoracentesis, headache following lumbar puncture, and anaphylaxis after intravenous contrast are adverse events.

When an adverse effect occurs, the system must undergo analysis to detect potential spots for improvement.

Preventable Adverse Event

This is an avoidable event in a particular set of circumstances.

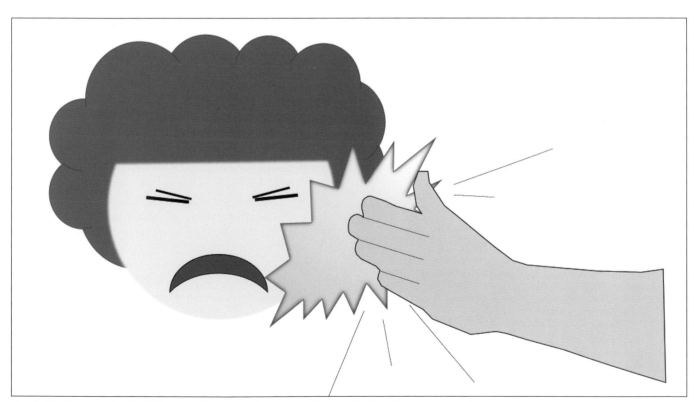

Fig. 1.10   Mnemonic SLLaP (System, Licensing, Liability, and Payment) of the four fundamental factors leading to errors.

Example: An infected central line as a result of poor sterile technique at the time of the line placement is a preventable adverse effect.

Tip: Not all errors result in harm. But they are still errors and must be treated as such.

James Reason

James Reason is a human error psychology expert. He notes that human error is a social label that implies that the individual should have acted differently and is therefore responsible. This is the basis of the "shame and blame" culture that has been so common in healthcare. Shame and blame is a roadblock to process improvement.[20]

If we understand the root causes of these human errors, and there are many, we should be able to improve. Some of these causes include communication failure, lack of effective training, memory lapses, inattention, poorly designed equipment, fatigue, ignorance, and noisy or distracting working conditions.

Example: Reading screening mammograms in a secluded batched format (away from noise and distractions) improves accuracy.

Malpractice

Quiz: You miss a large pneumothorax on a chest X-ray, and this blatant miss is clearly below the standard of care. However, the ER doctor catches it right away, places a chest tube, and cures the patient. Did you commit malpractice?

Answer: No. See below.

Error and malpractice are different. You might make a whopper of an error, but unless the following four criteria are established, that error does not constitute malpractice.[19]

The four criteria needed for malpractice include:

1. A doctor–patient relationship existed.
2. The doctor was negligent.
3. The doctor's negligence caused the injury.
4. The injury led to specific damages.

In addition, from a legal standpoint, the radiologist is generally obligated to meet the "standard of care," that is, what would the typical radiologist have done in the same situation?

Errors in detection are the most common cause of radiology malpractice suits. Other causes of malpractice suits include errors in interpretation, errors in communication of results, and errors in follow-up testing suggestions.

Radiology Errors

The two broad categories of error in radiology are perceptual and cognitive.[16]

Perceptual Error

The most common radiologist error is a *perceptual error*. This is a missed finding and accounts for 70% of our errors.

Example: A perceptual error is the pulmonary nodule that you see immediately when you are asked to review the case, but for some reason, you didn't see or dictate it the first time around. These errors are the hardest for us to accept.

Cognitive Error

The next most common radiologist error is a *cognitive error*. This error is the result of faulty interpretation of information. Secondary errors in the assessment of pretest probability, failure to seriously consider all relevant possibilities, and various forms of bias, may also contribute to cognitive errors.

Example: A cognitive error is the inappropriate further work-up of a clearly lipid-rich adrenal adenoma seen on a noncontrast CT, if you are not familiar with the criteria to definitively make that diagnosis.

Cognitive errors are more amenable to correction than are perceptual errors.

Other types of radiologist error include "treatment errors," "failure of communication," and "preventative errors." A prevention error might include inadequate screening of a patient with marginal renal function prior to administering iodinated contrast.

For any error, the first step in the response is the same, and that is to deal with the immediacy of the situation and the patient. However, the best response after that first step varies, depending upon the type of error.

Active and Sharp, Latent and Blunt
Active and Sharp

Say you read a right knee MRI, but report it as a left knee MRI. You are the final step in the radiology system, and your error is termed an *active error*. Errors like yours on the front lines occur at the "sharp end" of the process. The sharp end is the last line of defense against an error. This error occurs at points of contact between a human and some aspect of a larger system. Active errors are readily apparent and easy to blame.

Tip: Remember that the *sharp end* of the process is on the front lines, since a radiologist poking his needle into a patient is clearly working with a sharp end.

Latent and Blunt

Now say you are the MRI tech who delivered the hapless radiologist that same case. You scanned a right knee, but accidentally labeled it as a left knee. You have committed a *latent error*, and these errors occur at the "*blunt end*" of the process. The blunt end includes support for frontline workers (e.g., internal operational personnel, policy makers, and leaders). Blunt end staff decisions affect patient care, but less directly than do sharp end staff decisions. Latent errors are the result of decisions made far from the bedside that impact patient care. These decisions may include organizational flaws (e.g., staffing decisions based on fiscal motivations) or equipment errors that make the human and machine interface less than intuitive.[21]

Example: The referring doctor has trouble with the cumbersome new picture archives and communication system and enters the wrong diagnostic code. The radiologist, uninformed of the correct diagnosis, is not able to specifically address the diagnostic question.

Tip: Latent errors are "accidents waiting to happen."

Sentinel Event

A sentinel event is an unexpected occurrence involving death, serious injury, or risk thereof. A sentinel event is a big deal and signals the need for an immediate investigation and response. TJC takes these sentinel events very seriously.[22]

According to TJC, some of the most *frequent examples of sentinel events* include the following: delay in treatment, unintended retention of foreign body, operative/postoperative complication, suicide, fall, medication error, and "wrong patient, wrong site, wrong procedure." This last event is particularly common with interventional radiology.

Authority Gradient

This refers to the steepness of the command hierarchy. In general, a lower-level employee tends to be intimidated to speak up to or against a higher-level employee, even if that higher-level employee is making a mistake.

High authority gradients exist in most medical operations and impact negatively on safety.

Example: You and 10 other radiologists perform hysterosalpingograms (HSGs) at the same clinic, all with the same X-ray tech. You, for some reason, were not taught to close the plastic speculum at the time of removal from the patient's vagina. All of the other radiologists correctly close the speculum. The tech hears your patients complain about discomfort, but does not hear the other radiologists' patients complain. She correctly concludes that you are doing it wrong. However, she is intimidated by you and your position and chooses to ignore the problem. The result is that the procedural technique goes uncorrected and your patients continue to suffer.

Tip: High authority gradients undermine the safety culture as a result of underreported safety and quality problems.

SBAR

SBAR stands for "situation, background, assessment, and recommendation" and is a basic suggested communication framework that deals with an authority gradient. SBAR is largely used to help nurses and technologists frame discussions with doctors.[23]

The SBAR technique has become TJC's stated industry best practice for standardized communication in healthcare. Nurses or technologists are taught to report in concise narrative form.

Example: "Dr. Carducci, this is Howard, the MRI tech from the Eastern clinic."

Situation: "Here is the situation. We have patient Raj Agrawal for an MRI with gadolinium."

Background: "He has a creatinine of 1.8 and an estimated glomerular filtration rate (eGFR) of 39. His labs are stable since a month earlier. He is 67 and takes high blood pressure medication."

Assessment: "My assessment is that although he is at higher than average risk for developing renal problems, we still should be safe to give him the contrast."

Recommendation: "I recommend that we proceed with the gadolinium, but give extra hydration and decrease the injected dose. Do you agree?"

Disclosing an Error

What should you do when an error occurs? Over the past decade, it has become clear that the best course of action when an error occurs is to be honest with the patient and family.[29] Apologize, take the responsibility, and let them know exactly what steps will be taken to prevent similar events from occurring in the future. The very last thing you want is to appear as if you are trying to cover something up.

Tip: When an error occurs, definitely don't cover it up or alter the medical record.

Evaluate Risk and Adverse Events
Root Cause Analysis

There is a lot more to optimal safety than simply fixing the immediate problem and blaming the directly involved individual.

When an error occurs, it is necessary to play detective and identify the source of the problem. This process is called "root cause analysis" (RCA).

RCA is a tool used to identify active and latent errors. This creates a narrative of the event with a timeline.[24] This is also known as "systems analysis." The first step in RCA is the quick fix to the actual problem.

Example: Say you have a second patient in a two-day interval develop an anaphylactic reaction to the gadolinium injection. The first step is to save the patient. This first step doesn't solve the long-term problem.

The subsequent steps in RCA are to determine what could have caused something as rare as anaphylaxis to gadolinium to occur on consecutive days.

Tip: It is important with RCA to identify the system problems and avoid the trap of focusing on individuals' mistakes.

"Never Event"

According to the National Quality Forum, this is an easily preventable event of sufficient importance that should *never* occur in a properly functioning healthcare system. The appearance of a never event is a red flag that the system is likely flawed, and a full investigation is mandated by law.

Example: Arterial embolization performed on the wrong patient, or on the wrong side of the correct patient, is a never event. However, a large pneumothorax following thoracentesis does not qualify for this definition, since this is expected to happen in a very small percentage of patients.

Failure Mode and Effect Analysis (FMEA)

This is the process used to prospectively identify error in a system, assessing each step that can go wrong. This is somewhat subjective and typically used in chemical plants and nuclear power (less so in healthcare). Steps of FMEA include the following: Map out the process. Identify where things can go wrong. Estimate the probability that the failure will be detected. Estimate the consequence and severity. Use the data to produce a "criticality index."

Skill–Rule–Knowledge

The *Skill–Rule–Knowledge* classification of human error refers to the degree of the conscious control exercised by the individual over his or her activities.

Knowledge Error

Radiology example: Your ultrasound technologist doesn't quite understand that the significance between a hypoechoic and an anechoic breast lesion may be dramatic.

Real-life example: You are looking for a specific apartment building while driving. Since it is nighttime and raining, and because you are in an unfamiliar and crowded city, you get lost.

These examples are both "knowledge errors." They don't happen because someone is interrupted or working too fast. These mistakes occur because the unskilled users simply don't understand the process. Knowledge errors respond well to extra training.

Skill Error

Radiology example: A patient has a PET/CT that you report as negative. The patient then has a brain CT showing a metastatic lesion in the cerebellum. If you had changed the intensity of the brain on the PET images (which you usually do in your typical search pattern, but for some reason skipped this time), you would have noticed this metastatic focus on the PET.

Real-life example: You are driving on a freeway that you have taken 100 times. You always get off at the same exit, but this time you are deep into an important phone conversation and suddenly notice that you have missed your exit. This is a *slip or a lapse* and the type of error you make while on autopilot.

As noted previously, most errors in radiology fall into this category. Unlike a knowledge error, this type of error does not respond to more training. You already know everything you need to know about brain metastases, and you definitely know where that highway exit is located. This error is often caused by strong intrusions. Preventing intrusions, adding workflow checklists, creating redundancy, and having auto alerts can all help to minimize this source of error.

Rule Error

This error falls in between the other two.

Radiology example: You have developed standard reporting templates for a CT head and know exactly what verbiage is required to justify insurer reimbursement. However, the insurance company decides to change the rules, and now denies, "Altered level of consciousness" as a reimbursable code. "Altered mental status" is now the accepted verbiage. However, you are certain that the old way works, and you don't know about the new rules. With your "strong but wrong" mentality, you wind up with a bunch of nonreimbursed scans.

Tip: The assumption that "more training" is the right fix for all errors is not true. One key in preventing future error is choosing the right corrective method.

High-Reliability Organization

"*High-reliability organizations*" can and must operate in a high-stress, high-risk environment.[25] For example, aircraft carrier operators, firefighters, and the military fall into this category. Lucky us—so does medicine! When a code is called or when you are simply reading a PET/CT, lives are at stake. You can't afford to let the ultrasound tech asking you a question or both telephones on your desk ringing distract you from successfully completing your top priorities. Those of us working in this type of high-reliability organization must be at the top of our game, even when the stakes are raised and the emotions are flying.

Five high-reliability organization characteristics are as follows:

1. *Preoccupation with failure* (in a good way): This guarantees high vigilance and a low trigger to explore red flags. This also commits resources.
2. *Avoidance of oversimplification*: The battalion chief of the firefighters or the CEO of a hospital might tend to oversimplify problems, but the staff working on the front lines (who vividly experience those problems) won't permit that oversimplification. Frontline workers have the unique perspective to be able to explain the details to their superiors, so it is crucial to listen to them.
3. *Sensitivity to operations:* Everyone from bottom to top in the chain of command needs a voice in operations. Collaboration across the ranks must be encouraged.
4. *Respect of expertise:* The best person for the job must be permitted to do that job. Authority gradient challenges should be overcome.
5. *Dedication to resilience*: A great system understands that errors will happen and is ready for them when they do. Acknowledge high risk, commit to safety, and create a blame-free environment. When mistakes happen, take them seriously, but learn to roll with the punches.

Human Reliability Curve

Scholars note (and then plot on curves) that as system factors improve, human performance increases, but will never reach 100%. Errors are inevitable.

Culture

Safety Culture

A critical step in organizational improvement is adopting a *safety culture.*

This is a blame-free environment where individuals are free to report errors or near misses, without fear of reprimand or punishment.[26] This begins with the leadership but includes all employees. Communication is key and safety is always the top priority. In a safety culture, people pursue safety on a daily basis and take action when needed. This can sometimes be difficult, since pointing out blame to coworkers is often uncomfortable.

The Agency for Healthcare Research and Quality (AHRQ) has developed a patient safety culture survey to objectively measure the success of an organization's safety culture.

Just Culture

A safety culture is also complemented by a *just culture.* A *just culture* maintains individual accountability by establishing zero tolerance for reckless behavior.[27] A just culture distinguishes between human errors/slips, at-risk behavior, and reckless behavior.

Human Error/Slips

This is an inadvertent action, and often the result of current system design and individual behavioral choices.

Example: The portable intensive care unit X-ray just shot didn't get recorded because the inexperienced X-ray tech pushed the wrong button. This tech shouldn't be punished as if an intentional or reckless error had been committed. In fact, if the punishment is too severe for the "crime," the tech may feel the undeserved pangs of the "second victim syndrome." Human errors and slips should be managed through changes in design, procedures, and training. **Action: console.**

At-risk Behavior/Taking Shortcuts

This is an action where the person committing the error believes that the risk is justified. At-risk behavior is choosing to do something in a way that unintentionally imposes a chance for harm to occur.

Radiology example: Choosing to read mammograms on a non–Mammography Quality Standards Act and Program (MQSA)-approved monitor because all of the approved monitors are occupied is at-risk behavior.

Real life example: Driving above the speed limit is at-risk behavior.

At-risk behavior should be managed through removal of incentives for the behavior, creating better incentives, and improving situation awareness. **Action: coach.**

Reckless Behavior/Ignoring Required Safety steps

This is an action that knowingly puts someone in harm's way. The risk is identified but ignored.

Example: You are a teleradiologist and receive payment per case read. The only cases on the list are PET-CTs, for which you have no training. You know you should not read these cancer patients' scans, but since you want to make money, you slug through them anyway. This is a conscious disregard for a substantial and unjustifiable risk. This should be managed through punitive action. **Action: punish.**

Tip: Console, coach, or punish based on the crime, not the outcome. Even if nothing bad resulted, reckless behavior deserves consequences.

Human Factors Engineering

Is it really safer to make a hands-free phone call while driving than to make a call with a handheld device? Psychologists in the field of human factors engineering analyze this type of question. These researchers consider human strengths and limitations when designing interactive systems and tools for people.

Forcing Function

The most effective solution to human error is a *forcing function*. A forcing function is a human factors engineering design that prevents the wrong thing from happening. It basically "idiot proofs" the system component in question. Many problems are fixable with automation types of forcing function.

Medical example: Say a ward in the hospital needs complete quarantine because of a possible contagion. You could hang up a bunch of warning signs, but that doesn't guarantee that foolish people won't still wander in. However, physically locking the ward entrance does guarantee a successful quarantine.

Real-life example: Microwave ovens use a forcing function. The oven won't turn on until the door is closed.

Practice Communication

The ACR has developed practice guideline standards for the communication of diagnostic imaging findings.[28] Consider the following questions.

- What should you do if you can't reach the referring doctor, but there is a critical finding? For example, what if an outpatient brain MRI for headache shows an unexpected intracranial mass, and you conclude that the patient shouldn't be driving?
- Should curbside consults be documented?
- Are all of the following satisfactory methods of nonroutine communication: text, instant message, email, and voice message?
- Can your tech give the referring service a nonroutine communication on your behalf?
- Is the ACR guideline for the communication of diagnostic imaging findings a legally binding document?

Answers to all of these, along with key points of the ACR document, are discussed below.

The ACR Guidelines

This ACR practice parameter is not a legally binding document. But if you deviate significantly, you should probably document why.

An effective method of communication should promote patient care, support the ordering physician/healthcare provider, minimize the risk of communication errors, and be timely.

The Other Guys

There is a reciprocal duty of information exchange, which includes the referring service. Communication is not simply a one-way street.

An imaging request should contain relevant clinical information, a working diagnosis, pertinent clinical signs and symptoms, and ideally a specific question to be answered. All of this is up to them, and this may be out of your hands.

Your Report

First, a physician (not a tech, physician assistant, or registered physician assistant) must generate the report. The report should include patient demographics and relevant clinical information. Any significant patient reaction should be documented, follow-up or additional diagnostic studies should be suggested (when appropriate), and, unless very brief, the report should contain an "impression." The final report should be proofread, and abbreviations and acronyms limited, to avoid ambiguity. The report is a definitive document, in compliance with the appropriate regulations, transmitted to the ordering provider, and archived according to state and federal regulations.

Preliminary Reports

These may be either written or verbal and should become a part of the permanent record. Significant variation between preliminary and final reports should be promptly reported and documented.

Standard Communication

The interpreting physician should expedite delivery of the report in reasonable timeliness. This is usually delivered to the ordering physician and/or designees.

Informal Communication

We all encounter these sometimes challenging situations.

Example: Say the oncologist knows and trusts you and wants you to review a CT scan that your colleague read. This patient has a history of lung cancer, in remission, with a reported new renal mass. The oncologist wants to know if the mass is new, and if it is more likely metastatic or a separate new primary. To complicate matters, the only comparison he gives you is an outside report that did not describe a renal mass. This form of curbside consult, often in suboptimal conditions, carries inherent risk.

Tip: The key recommendation for informal interpretations is twofold: radiologists should document these interpretations and radiology groups should develop a formalized system for reporting outside studies.

Nonroutine Communication

Sometimes nonroutine communication is warranted. Indications may include the following:

- Findings needing immediate or urgent intervention (e.g., significantly misplaced lines, pneumothorax, or other deviations from the institution's critical value conditions)
- Findings discrepant with a preceding same patient interpretation, where failure to act may lead to an adverse outcome
- Findings serious enough that, if not acted on, may worsen over time and result in an adverse outcome (e.g., infectious process, malignant lesion)

Methods of Nonroutine Communication

Use a method that will most effectively reach the treating service, avoid a potential break in continuity of care, and maximally benefit the patient.

This communication should be made by telephone or in person. Other methods (text, fax, voice message, instant messaging, email) may not guarantee timely receipt, may not be Health Insurance Portability and Accountability Act of 1996 (HIPAA) compliant, and are not recommended.

This communication may be accomplished directly by the interpreting physician or, when judged appropriate, by the interpreting physician's designee. Your tech may give a result at your request.

When the referring service is unavailable, it may be appropriate to convey results directly to the patient.

Nonroutine Communication Documentation

This documentation is best placed in the patient's medical record or report. Another option is to document in a departmental log and/or personal journal.

The documentation should include the time, method of communication, and name of the person to whom the communication was delivered.

Tip: Document all nonroutine communications. If you didn't document, you didn't do it (at least legally).

Self-referred Patient

A self-referred patient establishes a doctor–patient relationship with the radiologist, and with that comes the responsibility for the radiologist to communicate findings directly to the patient.

Third-party Referrals

When patients are referred by third parties (insurance companies, employers, federal benefit programs, and lawyers), findings should be communicated to the third party, as the referrer. In certain situations, the radiologist may deem it appropriate and ethically correct to also communicate the findings directly to the patient.

Final ACR Points

The ACR advises radiology departments to develop written communication policies, which must be shared and followed. The ACR also recommends that all imaging reports be made readily available to the patient. This can be accomplished in various ways, including the posting of imaging reports through a web-based portal.

Swiss Cheese

Safety expert James Reason described the *Swiss cheese* model of accident causation. Organizations have many layers of defense, but none are foolproof, and all have holes. Sometimes these holes align, allowing the errors to result in patient harm.

Take the following fictional scenario and the "Swiss cheese"–type steps that transpired to result in a bad outcome.

Example Overview

A radiologist misses a small cavernous sinus meningioma on a CT head. This leads to a delay in diagnosis. When the mass is finally detected, the patient has lost vision in one eye. What went wrong?

First problem

The radiologist was slightly distracted. At the same time he was reading the study, he received an anxious call from the ER doctor needing him to quickly open up a "rule-out extravasation" trauma CT abdomen. The radiologist asked the ER doctor to hold on for just a second, while he "quickly finished up a head CT." The radiologist isn't usually asked to immediately look at an emergency case, but he was this time.

Second problem

The patient changed the order. The study was ordered with contrast. Although the patient had no contraindication, she decided to decline the contrast. The technologist later noted that the patient was somewhat rude and difficult to deal with. On the noncontrast study, the meningioma was isodense to brain (and difficult to see). Months later on the post contrast follow-up study, the meningioma was enhancing/hyperdense and easily detectable. A patient doesn't usually change the referring service order, but she did this time.

Third problem

Poor doctor–patient communication. The follow-up recommendations were not clearly conveyed during the ER doctor and patient discussion. The patient claims the ER did not specifically tell her to get a contrast study or MRI, if the symptoms persisted. The ER service usually is very careful to provide and

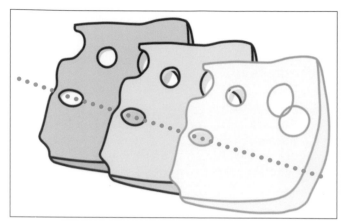

Fig. 1.11 Swiss-cheese–type error layers. Compound buildup of small errors leading to a large complication.

document follow-up recommendations, but perhaps because this patient was somewhat difficult to deal with, either the conversation or at least the documentation was neglected.

These Swiss cheese–type error layers unfortunately coordinated to permit the delay in diagnosis (**Fig. 1.11**).

Key Safety Goals

Key patient safety goals, per TJC.[30]

Use at Least Two Patient Identifiers Before Any Procedure

Satisfactory identifiers include the patient's name, date of birth, phone number, patient ID number, government–issued photo ID, and last four of the social security number. The patient's location or room number *cannot* be used.

Report Critical Results of Tests on a Timely Basis

Label all medications. In radiology, this includes medicines in syringes. Do this in the area where medicines and supplies are set up (**Fig. 1.12**).

Communicate Accurate Patient Information

Take extra care with patients who use blood thinners. Record and pass along correct information about a patient's medicine.

Prevent Infection

Use the hand-cleaning guidelines from the Center for Disease Control and Prevention (CDC) or the World Health Organization (WHO).

Prevent central line–associated bloodstream infections.

The Procedural Radiologist

The procedural radiologist, a qualified assistant (nurse practitioner or physician assistant), or the referring provider, should perform a specific patient assessment. The assessment should include the history and physical, risk assessment for sedation (if needed), and relevant preprocedure lab tests or other diagnostic tests.

Consent

Informed consent is required for all invasive and some non-invasive medical procedures.[31] Patients have the right to be informed about the procedures and may request to speak with the radiologist, even when local policy doesn't require the radiologist to actually obtain the informed consent.

Who Can Obtain the Consent?

This can be obtained by the healthcare provider performing the procedure or by another qualified person assisting the provider. Your tech or aid can obtain the consent. Note that the physician or other provider performing the procedure remains ultimately responsible for answering patient questions/concerns.

Who Can Give the Consent?

The patient should give consent (unless mentally incapable or has not reached the locally recognized age of majority). In those instances, or if the patient is otherwise not able to

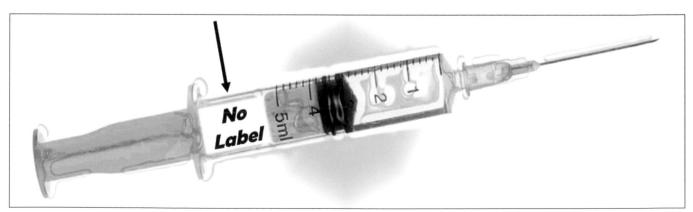

Fig. 1.12 Label all medications, including medicine in syringes.

give consent, permission may alternatively be given by a relative, guardian/legal representative, domestic partner, or healthcare provider who knows the patient.

What Must the Consent Include?

This informed consent must include a discussion of benefits, potential risks, reasonable alternatives to the procedure, and risks of refusing the procedure. Note that it is probably not reasonable to discuss *every* conceivable risk. This risk disclosure is a balance between reasonable consent and unreasonable alarmist information. For example, discussing the risk of death as a result of anaphylactic reaction from intravenous contrast is probably not necessary.

What About in an Emergency?

In an emergency situation, the medical staff may provide treatment without consent to "prevent serious disability or death or to alleviate great pain or suffering."

The Easiest Settlement

A friend of mine outside of work happens to be a malpractice attorney (…"Keep your friends close…"…right?) He told me the story of "the easiest settlement he ever had." Something went wrong during a medical procedure, and during the preliminary discovery it was noted that nobody had ever obtained the consent for the procedure. The doctors and staff had simply forgotten. Open and shut case for the plaintiff.

Tip: Trust no one and assume nothing. Double-check the consent.

Universal Preprocedural Verification Process
The three keys (Fig. 1.13)

1. *Confirm correct surgery on correct patient at correct body part.* Attempt to involve the patient in this confirmation. Additionally, identify the items needed for the procedure. Use a standard list to verify availability of the needed items, and then match these items to the patient.
2. *Mark the procedure site.* Use an unambiguous mark, which is preferably standardized throughout the organization. Only the person performing the exam, or a specific designee, should make the mark. The mark should be at or near the correct site and remain visible after prep and draping. The use of adhesive markers is not permitted. On occasion, a mark is not possible (i.e., on a mucosal surface), or advised (i.e., on the skin of an infant, who may be at risk for permanent stain/tattoo). In those cases, adhere to local policies.
3. *Perform a "time-out."* Time-out procedures are mandatory for all invasive procedures and for some noninvasive procedures. A time-out should be

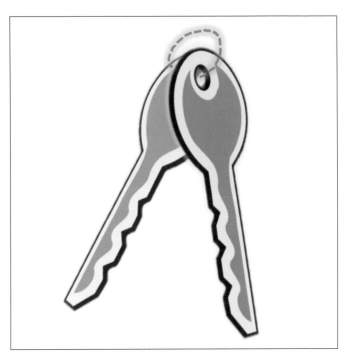

Fig. 1.13 Keys to universal preprocedural verification.

standardized and documented, and should occur just prior to the procedure. A designated team member should start the time-out, and all members of the team must share involvement and ultimately communicate and agree. The patient should be involved in the process, if he or she is able. If multiple procedures are planned for a given patient, multiple time-outs are required.

Medication reconciliation

This is the process of reviewing the patient's complete medication regimen at a point of transition and comparing it with the regimen being considered for the new setting of care. This should be done on admission, transfer, and discharge.

Six "rights"

Any time medication is administered, six elements must occur. The right medicine should be given to the right patient, via the right route, with the right dose, at the right time, and with the right documentation. This alliterative phrase constitutes the six "rights" of medication administration.

Simulation-Based Training

Simulation is a learning technique that replaces (or amplifies) real-life experiences with guided ones that replicate substantial aspects of the real world. This often takes place in an "immersive" fashion. In medicine, simulation-based learning can help develop healthcare professionals' skills, while protecting patients from unnecessary risks.[32]

Tip: "I hear and forget. I see and remember. I do and I understand."—Confucius (551–479 BC)

For example, we have all used simulation with training models associated with Advanced Cardiovascular Life Support (ACLS) and Basic Life Support (BLS) courses. There are a lot more examples in medicine. In addition to technical and functional training, simulation-based learning is useful for problem-solving, decision-making skills, and interpersonal skills. Some uses in radiology include virtual procedural stations (to practice image-guided biopsies), simulated clinical environments (to practice codes or contrast reaction scenarios), and electronic medical records (for staff to practice system integration or patient scheduling).

Not all simulation works or is optimally devised. Some considerations when assessing a simulation's effectiveness include: Are the simulated objects accurate reproductions? Is this particular subject amenable to simulation training? Does the simulation successfully teach what is required? Is there a better way to teach this subject instead of simulation? Does this simulation predict real-life performance?

Tip: Listen to Confucius. Incorporating simulation training in your practice—drilling code procedures, for example—adds another layer of understanding and safety.

Appropriateness Criteria

The ACR has developed appropriateness criteria and decision support. The purpose is to assist physicians in making good imaging decisions for various patient clinical situations.[33]

These criteria rely on the best evidence available, employ the input of radiologists and other medical specialists, and are posted on the National Guidelines Clearinghouse (NGC), a subset of the AHRQ. Topics include diagnostic radiology, interventional radiology, and radiation oncology.

Ten ACR appropriateness imaging criteria topics include breast, cardiac, gastrointestinal, musculoskeletal, neuro, pediatrics, thoracic, urologic, vascular, and women's imaging. Expert panels comprised of radiologists and clinical specialists outside of radiology maintain the topics, each of which contains various clinical conditions.

Each variant is scored on a 1–9 scale (1 = low, 9 = high).

- 1–3: test usually not appropriate.
- 4–6: test may be appropriate.
- 7–9: test usually appropriate.

Additionally, relative radiation risk is included for decision support.

Tip: Decision support use will be mandated by CMS for reimbursement in 2017.

Practice Parameters and Technical Standards

The ACR practice parameters and technical standards define principles and technical parameters and describe a range of acceptable approaches for diagnosis and treatment. These are reviewed at least every 5 years and allow for differences in training, experiences, and local conditions. Technical standards are quantitative or measureable and focus on physics and nuclear medicine.

Peer Review

Peer review is required by the ACR to ensure that ongoing quality review processes are in place. There is no punitive aspect, the process is anonymous, and peer review data are immune to legal action or discovery. A variety of biases may hamper the peer review process, and these should be avoided as much as possible.

TJC checks that a peer review process is ongoing but does not review the actual data.

RadPeeR

RadPeeR is a program that many radiology departments use for their peer review. Radiologists typically sample 5 to 10% of each other's cases. Specialists usually only rate other specialists, and the samples are random.

RadPeeR data is often conveniently linked to ongoing professional practice evaluation (OPPE) and focused provider practice evaluation (FPPE).

RadPeeR data are scored as follows:

1. Concur.
2. Discrepancy, but not ordinarily expected to be made. An understandable miss.
3. Discrepancy, and diagnosis should be made most of the time.
4. Discrepancy, and diagnosis should be made almost every time. A clear misinterpretation of the study.

Additionally, RadPeeR data 2, 3, and 4 are further subdivided into the following:

- Unlikely to be clinically significant.
- Likely to be clinically significant.

Tip: QI data are not discoverable in a court of law.

Miscellaneous Organizations Contributing to Quality and Safety

ACR: RadPeeR, modality certification, practice guidelines, and technical standards, BI-RADS (LI-RADS, PI-RADS, etc.), and appropriateness criteria.

American Roentgen Ray Society (ARRS): educational courses, Practice Quality Improvement (PQI) projects.

Radiologic Society of North America (RSNA): quality storyboards, PQI projects.

Agency for Healthcare Research and Quality (AHRQ): government agency, part of Health and Human Services.

Institute for Healthcare Improvement (IHI): organization dedicated to improve healthcare worldwide.

National Quality Forum (NQF): reported on "Never Events."

The Joint Commission (TJC): required for licensure. May audit without warning.

Nuclear Regulatory Commission (NRC): licenses and radiation safety.

Magnetic Resonance Imaging Safety

Quiz: If a patient codes while in the scanner, should you press the quench button (which turns off the magnet) so that you can safely initiate BLS in the scanner room?

Answer: No. If there is a cardiac arrest in the MR suite, immediately move the patient to a magnetically safe location (Zone 3 or lower), and then initiate BLS.

Why Not Press Quench?

Every MR suite has a red button on the wall for quenching (and a quench turns off the magnet). However, a quench also causes dangerous room heating and release of noxious gases. In addition, a completed quench is not instantaneous. It might take a couple of minutes, and seconds count in a code situation.

When Should You Press Quench?

If there is a metal-related dangerous situation (e.g., an oxygen tank has smashed into the gantry and injured a patient), then quenching is the correct option. During a quench, make sure to evacuate the room because of the dangers described above.

To minimize the significant ferromagnetic safety risks of the MR scanner magnet, special mandated precautions exist for every MRI department.[34] There are four zones and they are all color-coded. Zone 1 (green) is the safest and most removed from the magnet. Zone 4 (red) is actually in the MRI room.

The four MR safety zones are as follows:

* Zone 1: outside (green)
* Zone 2: nearby, but no door to MRI suite (blue)
* Zone 3: nearby, with door to MRI suite (yellow)
* Zone 4: room housing the MRI (red)

Contrast Allergies and Reactions

The two main challenges associated with iodinated contrast administration are contrast-related allergies and contrast-induced nephropathy (CIN).[35]

Incidence

The incidence of any contrast reaction is 0.2 to 0.7%. The incidence of a severe reaction with low osmolality contrast is 0.01 to 0.02%. The greatest risk factor for a reaction is a history of a prior contrast reaction. This increases the risk of subsequent reaction fivefold. However, even in a patient with a history of prior reaction, and without the addition of a pretreatment regimen, the risk of subsequent reaction is still less than 10%.

Shellfish, Asthma, and Atopic Patients

Atopic patients have a twofold to threefold increased risk of reaction. Asthmatic patients may also have a slightly increased risk. Shellfish allergy patients have an equivocal increased risk of contrast reaction.

Premedication

Prednisone: 50 mg PO 13 hours, 7 hours, and 1 hour prior. Diphenhydramine (Benadryl): 25 to 50 mg intravenous (IV)/intramuscular (IM) or PO 1 hour prior.

Tip: Note that IV steroids are not effective when administered less than 4 to 6 hours prior to contrast.

What can premedication accomplish?

Premedication is proven to reduce the incidence of minor reactions. Premedication is not proven to protect against severe life-threatening injuries, although the rarity of severe reactions makes it difficult to study this question. For practical purposes, if a patient has a history of a severe reaction (and if after careful risk–benefit assessment, the decision is made to administer contrast), a premedication regimen is recommended.

Breakthrough reactions

Some patients will exhibit breakthrough reactions despite premedication. These reactions are most often similar to the index reaction. If these patients are subsequently premedicated, the large majority won't have another breakthrough reaction. Patients with a mild index reaction have an extremely low risk of subsequently developing a severe breakthrough reaction. Severe allergies to any other substance are associated with a somewhat higher risk of developing a moderate or severe breakthrough reaction.

Tip: Anaphylactic reactions are unpredictable and life-threatening.

Treating the Radiology Patient with a Contrast Reaction

Mild reaction

If a patient develops urticaria from contrast, no specific treatment is usually indicated. (Discontinue the injection if not already completed.) Benadryl improves the urticaria but also causes mild sedation.

Tip: Any patient with a mild reaction should be observed for at least 20 to 30 minutes, since mild reactions may evolve into more severe reactions.

More-Serious Reactions (Fig. 1.14)
Bronchospasm

Give oxygen 6 to 10 L/min via mask. Monitor electrocardiogram (EKG), oxygen saturation, and blood pressure. Give β-agonist inhaler (i.e., albuterol 2–3 puffs, when necessary). If there is no response, give epinephrine.

Give epinephrine subcutaneous (SC) or intramuscular (IM) (1:1,000) 0.1 to 0.3 mL (0.1–0.3 mg) or, especially if hypotension is evident, epinephrine 1:10,000 slowly intravenous (IV) 1–3 mL. Repeat as needed up to a maximum of 1 mg.

Hypotension with tachycardia

Elevate legs 60 degrees or more (or Trendelenburg, which is 15–30 degrees of legs higher than the head). Give oxygen 6 to 10 L/min via mask. Monitor EKG, oxygen saturation, and blood pressure. Bolus rapid IV large volume of lactated Ringer's or normal saline. If the response is poor, give epinephrine 1:10,000 slowly IV 1 mL (0.1 mg). Repeat as needed up to a maximum of 1 mg.

Hypotension with bradycardia (vagal)

Same initial steps as above, but instead of epinephrine, if poorly responsive, give atropine 0.6 to 1 mg IV slowly. Repeat up to a total dose of 0.4 mg/kg (2–3 mg) in an adult.

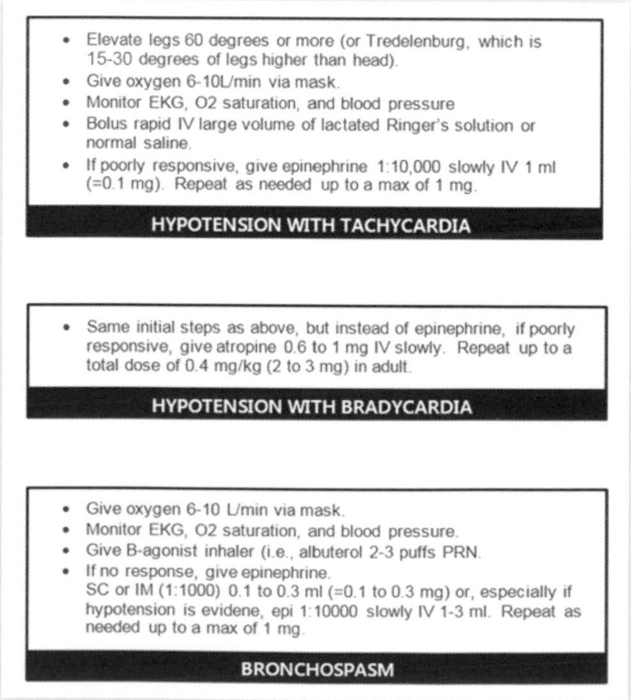

Fig. 1.14 Treating patients with contrast reactions.

Physiologic but Undesirable Effects

These include arrhythmias, depressed myocardial contractility, cardiogenic pulmonary edema, functional hypocalcemia, and even seizures. Contrast problems are often dose and concentration dependent. It is reasonable to consider slightly lowering the dose in a higher-risk patient.

Contrast Nephropathy

This is defined as the impairment of renal function attributable to recent contrast administration. There is some debate on the standard criteria, but many make this diagnosis when there is a 25% increase in serum creatinine from baseline, or a 0.5 mg/dL increase in absolute value, within 48 to 72 hours of intravenous contrast administration. Creatinine levels typically peak within 2 to 5 days and revert to normal within 7 to 10 days. The development of permanent renal dysfunction is rare, but there does appear to be a (complex) relationship between CIN, additional morbidity, and even mortality.

Risk Factors

Age, chronic kidney disease (CKD), diabetes, hypertension (HTN), metabolic syndrome, anemia, multiple myeloma, hypoalbuminemia, renal transplant, hypovolemia, and decreased left ventricular ejection fraction (LVEF) are all risk factors. Low osmolality contrast is less nephrotoxic than high osmolality contrast. Cardiac procedures result in a much higher incidence of CIN than do diagnostic radiology procedures.

Prevention

Giving IV fluids before contrast administration is the most proven method of reducing risk. One suggestion is to begin hydration 6 hours prior to contrast and continue for 6–24 hours afterward. Congestive heart failure and other fluid-intolerant patients pose a special challenge.

A variety of other pretreatment regimens, including mannitol, lasix, theophylline, endothelin-1, and fenoldopam, are less proven, and use of these agents for the prevention of CIN is *not* recommended.

Using a lower dose of contrast may be helpful. Most authors agree to keep the contrast dose less than 100 mL, since studies have shown that the need for subsequent dialysis when contrast is kept to that dose or lower is very rare.

For a patient with a moderate to severe risk of CIN, the estimated glomerular filtration rate (eGFR) should be estimated precontrast and then remeasured 24 to 48 hours postcontrast. If CIN develops, hydration is the cornerstone of therapy.

Tip: The best treatment for CIN is prevention. Screen appropriately, use the lowest dose of contrast possible, and ensure IV hydration.

Quiz: Is taking metformin a risk factor for developing CIN?

Answer: No, but a patient with renal failure while taking metformin is at risk for developing lactic acidosis.

The Story with Metformin

This oral diabetes medicine can result in a dangerous build-up of lactic acid, but only if the contrast medium causes renal dysfunction and the patient continues to take the metformin. The safest way to approach these patients is to have them withhold their metformin for 48 hours after contrast administration. (They will likely need to contact their referring physician to make alternative glucose management plans during this time.) If normal and stable creatinine is subsequently confirmed at 48 hours, the metformin may then be safely restarted.

MRI and Gadolinium

A true allergy to MR contrast agents is very rare (reported incidence 0.004–0.7%). Life-threatening reactions are even more rare (0.001–0.01%). Despite the rarity, problems do occur, and on-site staffing to monitor MR contrast is always mandated.

Gadolinium and Nephrogenic Systemic Fibrosis

Use of gadolinium-based contrast medium in patients with moderate chronic kidney disease (CKD) and an eGFR of less than 30 mL/min has been implicated in the development of nephrogenic systemic fibrosis (NSF), a chronic debilitating illness with no cure.

The major risk factor for developing NSF is end-stage CKD (Stage 5, eGFR < 15 mL/min) or severe CKD (Stage 4, eGFR between 15 and 29 mL/min). Stage 4 patients have a 1 to 7% chance of developing NSF after one or more exposures. Most patients who develop NSF are already on dialysis.

There has only been one published report of a patient with an eGFR > 30 mL/min developing NSF.

Other risk factors for NSF include the use of higher doses and multiple doses of gadolinium, currently receiving dialysis, and acute kidney injury.

Recommendation

If the eGFR < 30 mL/min, do not administer gadolinium. If the eGFR is between 30 and 45 mL/min, it is probably safe to administer, but use the following to shape your final decision. Is the eGFR stable or falling? Is the patient on dialysis? Has there been a recent renal insult? If the answer to all three questions is no, it is likely safe to administer contrast.

Tip: To prevent NSF, screen appropriately. Use the lowest dose of contrast possible and ensure hydration.

What About the Fetus?

No adverse effects to the fetus have been documented after a pregnant woman has received gadolinium. However, there is the theoretical risk of potential dissociation of gadolinium. (This is also the proposed mechanism for the formation of NSF.) So, gadolinium is relatively contraindicated in the pregnant patient.

Quiz: Should a patient discontinue breastfeeding after receiving gadolinium? How about for iodinated contrast?

Answer: No for both. While it is true that very small amounts of both contrast agents have been detected in breast milk, this extremely small volume is considered safe.

Extravasation

The tech enters the reading room with the bad news that there has been a contrast extravasation. Despite shrinking down into your comfortable chair, trying to go unnoticed, the tech selects you for help. What do you do?

Quiz: Which is more effective in treating contrast extravasation: warm compresses or cold compresses?

Answer: Trick question. There is no clear evidence to favor the superiority of either. Both are reasonable options.

Risk Factors

These are risk factors for both contrast extravasation and for increasing volume of extravasated contrast: inability of the patient to communicate, severe illness, abnormal limb circulation, distally positioned venous access site, multiple punctures in the same vein, and the use of an indwelling line for greater than 24 hours.

Tip: Although the *frequency* of extravasation is probably not related to the injection flow rate, the *severity* of the extravasation is likely greater with a power injector.

Most patients have no significant sequelae from extravasation. However, each patient needs assessment, since prompt medical attention is mandated if complications do occur.

Complications

Compartment syndrome and skin necrosis are the main two potential complications of extravasation. The risk of compartment syndrome increases as the volume of contrast increases. Tissue necrosis may occur since extravasated contrast is toxic to skin and the surrounding soft tissues. This risk of necrosis increases in patients with arterial compromise, poor venous drainage, or poor lymphatic drainage.

Treatment of Contrast Extravasation

Elevate the extremity. Either warm or cold compresses are reasonable treatments. There is no clear evidence to support attempting aspiration of the contrast.

Contrast Warming

Contrast media viscosity decreases with increasing temperature. Warming contrast media from room temperature to body temperature decreases viscosity and decreases resistance during the injection. Both of these are desirable effects and may result in improved vascular opacification. This is especially apparent and/or important in the following circumstances: with higher flow rate injections, when utilizing higher viscosity contrast agents, for direct arterial injections through small caliber catheters, and when timing of the bolus and peak enhancement are critical.

To warm the contrast, most institutions use an external incubator kept at or near 37°C. In addition to these warming devices, warming sleeves are used to keep prewarmed bottles, or syringes from prewarmed bottles, warm for about an hour.

Since contrast media are considered to be medications, TJC has jurisdiction and mandates keeping a daily log and documenting regular maintenance for each warming device. This has proven to be a deterrent for some institutions to warm their contrast.

Studies have raised the possibility that warming iodinated contrast may reduce the incidence of mild contrast reactions or extravasation, but this has not been conclusively demonstrated.

Note that gadolinium is given at room temperature and should *not* be externally warmed.

Tip: For CT, warm the iodinated contrast. For MRI, do not warm the gadolinium contrast.

Radiation Safety

We have come a long way with radiation safety since Mrs. Roentgen first put her hand in front of a cathode ray tube. There are now a number of thoughtful radiation safety programs.[36]

Radiation Programs

Image Gently

This was initially produced by the Society of Pediatric Radiology, with the goal of raising awareness and minimizing radiation doses in pediatrics. The first focus was on children and their CT scans.

Step Lightly

This was initially introduced by pediatric interventional radiologists, who provided educational resources to further the goal of decreasing fluoroscopic doses. There are three phases with this program: Phase 1 educates the radiologists, technologists, and physicists. Phase 2 educates the referring services. Phase 3 educates the parents and public.

Image Wisely

This is the adult counterpart of Image Gently and was formed by the RSNA and the ACR. The focus is twofold: one, optimizing protocols and appropriate use of imaging, and two, communicating with patients, the public, and the medical community. The primary focus thus far has been with CT scans.

Patients are now able to track their exams and cumulative radiation doses with individual "patient medical imaging records."

Considerations When Explaining Radiation Risks to Patients

First of all, it is important to ensure that the exam is appropriate. It is also important to place context in the patient's diagnosis. Discussion of risk of the exam should also include the risk of not performing the exam. It is often a good idea to compare radiation risk to other radiation risk exposures (e.g., the radiation exposure for traveling in an airplane at 30,000 feet compared to the radiation exposure for the radiology test in question). Try to explain to the patient that risks are discussed in terms of populations and that individual risk, although obviously desired, is very difficult to determine.

CT Dose Index

This is a standardized measure of radiation dose output of a given CT scanner. This permits comparison with the radiation output from other CT scanners. Note that the CT dose index is a dose estimate and does not give the actual dose received by the patient. (The dose received depends on multiple factors including the CT scanner, technical parameters, scan protocol, number of phases, pitch, and tissue composition, size, and frequency. Medical physicists can calculate an estimated dose based on parameters of the study and specific patient factors.)

There are two main parameters calculated and reported by CT scanners:

1. *CTDI vol*: Volume-based CT dose index (units: mGy).
2. *DLP:* Dose-length product (units: mGy-cm). Note that DLP = CTDI vol × scan length (for helical scanning).

American College of Radiology: Dose Index Registry

Data of CTDI vol and DLP for CT scans performed are tracked and compared to those of other institutions. Facilities may use this data to track their own performance and adjust protocols.

The ACR has provided several reference CTDI vol values. These values let practices know whether their numbers are at least "in the ballpark":

- 75 mGy for a head CT
- 25 mGy for an adult abdomen CT
- 20 mGy for a pediatric abdomen CT

ALARA

Most of us are familiar with ALARA (as low as reasonably achievable).

Some key elements of ALARA include the following:

- Perform an exam only when it is indicated. If possible, consider ultrasound (USN) or MRI as nonionizing radiation imaging alternatives.
- Use the lowest dose techniques to obtain images. Modify current (mA) and tube potential (kV) for patient size.
- Use a lower kV for smaller patients when using iodinated contrast.
- Minimize multiphase protocols.
- Limit the length of long axis scanning.
- Document the dose in the medical record (for fluoroscopy and CT).

Five Test Indications that Should Be Questioned

According to the ACR, when "Choosing Wisely," the following *test indications should be questioned* and probably not performed:

1. No imaging for uncomplicated headache.
2. No imaging for low pretest probability of pulmonary embolism. This would include a negative D-dimer.
3. No pre-op CXR for a patient with an unremarkable history and physical exam. (CXR is probably reasonable if the patient has acute cardiopulmonary disease, or is older than 70 years, has chronic stable cardiopulmonary disease, and has had no CXR within the past 6 months.)
4. No CT for suspected appendicitis in a child without first at least considering USN.
5. No follow-up ultrasound for inconsequential adnexal cysts (e.g., classic corpus luteum cyst measuring less than 5 cm, 1 cm or smaller simple cyst in a postmenopausal woman).

Professionalism and Ethics

The Health Insurance Portability and Accountability Act of 1996 (HIPPA) required the U.S. Department of Health and Human Services (HHS) to adopt national standards for electronic healthcare transactions and code sets, unique health identifiers, and security. Congress subsequently mandated the adoption of federal privacy protections for individually identifiable health information.

Authorization not required. The following are situations for which individual authorization is "not" required for transfer of data: fraud or abuse detection, domestic violence or neglect, payment, quality of competency assurance, compliance activities, oversight agencies, judicial and administrative proceedings, law enforcement purposes, and worker's compensation cases.

Statistics

Sensitivity

The proportion of people who have the disease and test positive for it.[37]

A test with a high sensitivity is most useful for ruling out disease.

You can remember this by SNOUT: Use the test of SeNsitivity to rule OUT disease (**Fig. 1.15**).

For example, a chest CT has a very high sensitivity for the detection of a pulmonary nodule. If no nodule is detected, it is very unlikely that the patient has a pulmonary nodule.

Specificity

The proportion of people who do not have the disease and test negative for it.

A test with a high specificity is most useful for ruling in the disease.

You can remember this by SPIN: Use the test of SPecificity to rule IN disease (**Fig. 1.16**).

For example, a lower extremity Doppler ultrasound has a very high specificity for the detection of a blood clot. If a clot is detected, it is very likely that the patient indeed has a clot.

Positive Predictive Value (PPV)

The proportion of people with positive test results who actually have the disease (TP = true positive; FP = false positive):

$$PPV = TP/(TP + FP).$$

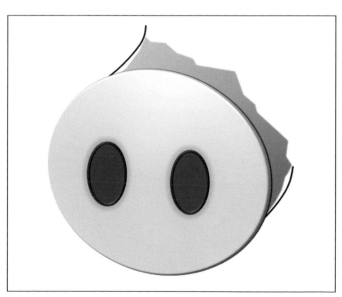

Fig. 1.15 Sensitivity testing. Use the test of SeNsitivity to rule OUT disease (SNOUT).

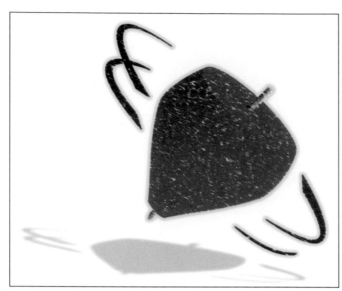

Fig. 1.16 Specificity testing. Use the test of SPecificity to rule IN disease (SPIN).

Negative Predictive Value (NPV)

The proportion of people with negative test results who do not have the disease (TN = true negative; FN = false negative):

NPV = TN/(TN+ FN).

One way to avoid confusing PPV and NPV is to imagine that you are a patient and have just received a positive test result. What is the probability that you really have the disease (i.e., how worried should you be)? If the positive predictive value is high, then you should be worried. The converse thinking is used with NPV.

Accuracy

The sum of TP and TN divided by the total number of subjects studied.

Precision versus Accuracy

Accuracy is how close a measured value is to the actual (true) value. Precision is how close the measured values are to each other (i.e., how much variation exists with repeated measurements).

One example of precision and accuracy is the utility of camera-based scintigraphy in nuclear medicine to determine the GFR. This method is considered precise but not accurate. Here, determining the absolute GFR is difficult. Since the scan has good precision, however, serial scanning is effective in assessing whether the unknown GFR is getting better or worse.

Tip: Something that is precise could be precisely wrong every time.

Memory tip:
- aCcurate is Correct.
- pRecise is Repeatable.

Receiver Operating Characteristic Curves

These curves plot the "sensitivity" versus "1-specificity." The "sensitivity" is the *y*-axis and is also known as the true-positive rate. "1-specificity" is the *x*-axis and is also known as the false-positive rate. The closer the receiver operating characteristic (ROC) curve is to the upper left-hand corner, the higher the overall accuracy of the test. A test with perfect discrimination (no overlap in the two distributions) has a right angle ROC curve that actually passes through the upper left corner (100% specificity and sensitivity). A straight 45-degree positive slope diagonal line represents a 50:50 test. The flip of a coin would yield the same results.

Quiz: How does prevalence of disease affect these numbers?

Answer: A critical concept is that the sensitivity, specificity, and the ROC curve (which is a graphical representation of the sensitivity and specificity) are intrinsic properties of a test and do not depend on the population being tested.

However, PPV, NPV, and accuracy are all affected by disease prevalence. The more rare the condition, the more likely a negative test is truly negative, and the less likely a positive test is truly positive.

Memory tip: If a statistic is affected by disease prevalence, you will constantly need to recalculate the results. That makes you very tired, so you will need a *NAP* (NPV, Accuracy, and PPV).

Radiology Error and Bias
Satisfaction of Search

This source of error occurs when the radiologist identifies a finding and then stops searching, even though another important abnormality is also present. This term is used in other fields but was actually first described for radiology.

Other Sources of Bias

There are many potential sources of error in statistical analysis, and a variety of biases contribute to these errors.[38]

- *Selection bias* occurs when data for analysis are compiled in such a manner that proper randomization is not achieved.
- *Spectrum bias*, a subtype of selection bias, occurs when the sample is missing important subgroups.
- *Verification bias* occurs when the results of a diagnostic test affect whether the gold standard procedure will be used to verify the test result.

- *Sampling bias* occurs if some members of the population are either more or less likely to be included in the study.
- *Measurement bias* occurs when methods of measurement are dissimilar between different groups of patients.
- *Review bias*, a subtype of measurement bias, occurs when tests are performed or interpreted without proper blinding.
- *Confounding bias* occurs when two factors are associated and the effect of one is distorted or confused by the effect of the other.
- *Lead-time bias* occurs when a new test merely identifies the disease earlier than did the previous test, thus giving the impression that the survival is longer. (An appropriate way to avoid lead-time bias is to compare age-specific mortality rates, rather than survival rates from the time of diagnosis.)
- *Length-time bias* occurs when screening tests falsely appear to improve survival, since they often detect more slowly growing diseases, which tend to have a better prognosis.
- *Screening bias* occurs because patients who volunteer for screening studies tend to be healthier and have better outcomes than nonvolunteers.
- *Overdiagnosis bias* occurs when screening identifies an illness that would not have shown clinical signs before a person's death from other causes.
- *Pygmalion effect bias* occurs when higher expectations lead to an increase in performance.

Tip: Consider the methodology validity, or flaws, when critically analyzing any scientific result. As radiologists, we are better equipped than the mainstream population to assess researchers' conclusions that reach the media.

Example: Much of the controversy regarding the best age to begin screening women with mammography involves various statistical biases.

Special Effects: Hawthorne and Weber

Hawthorne Effect

You are driving on an open highway when a police car pulls up behind you. What do you do? If you are like most people, you reflexively step on the brake a little while you quickly check your speed.

This is the Hawthorne effect. Simple awareness that you are being observed changes your behavior.

The Hawthorne effect was first described in the workplace.[39] A series of experiments was performed at the Chicago AT&T Hawthorne factory in the 1920s. Initially, workers were told that they would be exposed to greater light and that their subsequent productivity would be observed. Indeed, their productivity improved—briefly. But the change in productivity wasn't the result of better lighting. In fact, the experimenters found that *any* variable change in the workplace, including break schedules, working hours, or self-selection of nearby coworkers (as long as the workers knew they were being observed) resulted in improved productivity. These effects were all temporary. Further, researchers found that social factors (e.g., working as a team, choosing one's own coworkers, and perceived interest that the manager had in a project) were at least as important as physical improvements in working conditions on improving productivity.

Knowledge of these effects has had great applications in management. For research, the Hawthorne effect is one of the hardest biases to eliminate from an experiment.

Weber Effect

Adverse event reporting tends to increase in the first two years after introduction of a new agent or use for a new indication, peaks at the end of the second year, and then declines.[40] This pattern was first described in 1984 in the United Kingdom for a single drug and is known as the Weber effect. The Food and Drug Administration and other agencies have made concerted efforts to improve methods and reporting. Today, this effect is probably not as common. The Weber effect explains why in a PDSA cycle the incidence of an adverse event may initially rise.

Now turn to the next chapter for additional new material and to begin the question and answer format.

References

1. CMS.gov. https://www.cms.gov/research-statistics-data-and-systems/statistics-trends-and-reports/nationalhealthexpenddata/nhe-fact-sheet.html. Published 2015. Accessed May 6, 2016
2. HRSA.gov. http://www.hrsa.gov/quality/toolbox/methodology/qualityimprovement/. Published 2015. Accessed May 6, 2016
3. National Academies. http://www.nationalacademies.org/hmd/. Published 2016. Accessed May 6, 2016
4. American Board of Medical Specialties. http://www.abms.org/board-certification/a-trusted-credential/based-on-core-competencies/. Published 2016. Accessed May 6, 2016
5. Techtarget. http://searchsoftwarequality.techtarget.com/definition/best-practice. Published 2016. Accessed May 6, 2016
6. Techtarget. http://searchbusinessanalytics.techtarget.com/definition/business-intelligence-dashboard. Published 2016. Accessed May 6, 2016
7. Ettorchi-Tardy A, Levif M, Michel P. Benchmarking: a method for continuous quality improvement in health. Health Policy 2012;7(4):e101–e119
8. Porter ME. What is value in healthcare? N Engl J Med 2010;363(26):2477–2481
9. Klipfolio. https://www.klipfolio.com/resources/kpi-examples. Published 2015. Accessed May 6, 2016
10. Institute for Healthcare Improvement. http://www.ihi.org/resources/Pages/HowtoImprove/default.aspx. Published 2016. Accessed May 6, 2016
11. Lawal AK, Rotter T, Kinsman L, et al. Lean management in healthcare: definition, concepts, methodology and effects reported (systematic review protocol). Syst Rev 2014;3:103

12. Six Sigma Online. http://www.sixsigmaonline.org/six-sigma-training-certification-information/lean-six-sigma-wastes-and-principles/. Published 2015. Accessed May 6, 2016

13. American Society for Quality. http://asq.org/learn-about-quality/six-sigma/overview/overview.html. Published 2015. Accessed May 6, 2016

14. American Society for Quality. http://asq.org/learn-about-quality/six-sigma/overview/dmaic.html. Published 2015. Accessed May 6, 2016

15. American Society for Quality. http://asq.org/learn-about-quality/seven-basic-quality-tools/overview/overview.html. Published 2015. Accessed May 6, 2016

16. Sabih DE, Sabih A, Sabih Q, Khan AN. Image perception and interpretation of abnormalities; can we believe our eyes? Can we do something about it? Insights Imaging 2011;2(1):47–55

17. The National Academies of Sciences Engineering and Medicine. https://www.nationalacademies.org/hmd/Reports/1999/To-Err-is-Human-Building-A-Safer-Health-System.aspx. Published 2016. Accessed May 6, 2016

18. Grissinger M. Too many abandon the "second victims" of medical errors. P T 2014;39(9):591–592

19. Bal BS. An introduction to medical malpractice in the United States. Clin Orthop Relat Res 2009;467(2):339–347

20. Reason J. Human error: models and management. BMJ 2000;320(7237):768–770

21. Agency for Healthcare Research and Quality. https://psnet.ahrq.gov/primers/primer/21/systems-approach. Published 2015. Accessed May 6, 2016

22. The Joint Commission. http://www.jointcommission.org/sentinel_event.aspx. Published 2016. Accessed May 6, 2016

23. Safer Healthcare. http://www.saferhealthcare.com/sbar/what-is-sbar/. Published 2015. Accessed May 6, 2016

24. American Society for Quality. http://asq.org/learn-about-quality/root-cause-analysis/overview/overview.html. Published 2015. Accessed May 6, 2016

25. The Joint Commission. http://www.jointcommission.org/assets/1/6/chassin_and_loeb_0913_final.pdf. Published 2016. Accessed May 6, 2016

26. United States Department of Labor. https://www.osha.gov/SLTC/etools/safetyhealth/mod4_factsheets_culture.html. Published 2016. Accessed May 6, 2016

27. Boysen PG II. Just culture: a foundation for balanced accountability and patient safety. Ochsner J 2013;13(3):400–406

28. American College of Radiology. http://www.acr.org/Quality-Safety/Standards-Guidelines. Published 2016. Accessed May 6, 2016

29. Agency for Healthcare Research and Quality. https://psnet.ahrq.gov/primers/primer/2/error-disclosur3. Published 2015. Accessed May 6, 2016

30. The Joint Commission. http://www.jointcommission.org/standards_information/npsgs.aspx. Published 2016. Accessed May 6, 2016

31. The Joint Commission. http://www.jointcommission.org/assets/1/23/Quick_Safety_Issue_Twenty-One_February_2016.pdf. Published 2016. Accessed May 6, 2016

32. Al-Elq AH, Al-Elk. Simulation-based medical teaching and learning. J Family Community Med 2010;17(1):35–40

33. American College of Radiology. http://www.acr.org/Quality-Safety/Appropriateness-Criteria. Published 2016. Accessed May 6, 2016

34. American College of Radiology. http://www.acr.org/quality-safety/radiology-safety/mr-safety. Published 2016. Accessed May 6, 2016

35. American College of Radiology. http://www.acr.org/quality-safety/resources/contrast-manual. Published 2016. Accessed May 6, 2016

36. American College of Radiology. http://www.acr.org/quality-safety/radiology-safety/radiation-safety. Published 2016. Accessed May 6, 2016

37. Parikh R, Mathai A, Parikh S, Chandra Sekhar G, Thomas R. Understanding and using sensitivity, specificity and predictive values. Indian J Ophthalmol 2008;56(1):45–50

38. Sica GT. Bias in research studies. Radiology 2006;238(3):780–789

39. McCambridge J, Witton J, Elbourne DR. Systematic review of the Hawthorne effect: new concepts are needed to study research participation effects. J Clin Epidemiol 2014;67(3):267–277

40. Hoffman KB, Dimbil M, Erdman CB, Tatonetti NP, Overstreet BM. The Weber effect and the United States Food and Drug Administration's Adverse Event Reporting System (FAERS): analysis of sixty-two drugs approved from 2006 to 2010. Drug Saf 2014;37(4):283–294

2   Questions and Answers

Select one of the following for questions 1 through 4:

A. Bundling
B. CPT Codes
C. ICD-9
D. GPCI

Question 1. Which of the above refers to episodes of care when the individual components of a procedure are combined into one code for the purposes of billing?

Question 2. Which of the above is designed to provide uniform language information about medical services and procedures for physicians, coders, patients, and accrediting organizations?

Question 3. Which of the above is a code which has at least three digits and can be modified by a fourth?

Question 4. Concordance between which two items above often defines medical necessity?

Answers:

1—**A**: Another term for this is episode-based payments. In other words, payments are linked for multiple individual clinical services that beneficiaries receive during an episode of care. This potentially provides higher quality and more coordinated care at a lower cost to Medicare.

2—**B**: CPT stands for Current Procedural Terminology and is a registered trademark of the American Medical Association (AMA). CPT is the most widely accepted nomenclature for reporting medical services and procedures for both public and private health insurance.

3—**C**: ICD stands for International Classification for Diseases, and "9" represents the ninth edition. This is a medical classification list, agreed upon at an international conference by the World Health Organization (WHO), and copyrighted by the WHO. This list contains codes for diseases, signs and symptoms, abnormal findings, complaints, social circumstances, and external causes of injury or diseases. These standardized codes help to improve consistency in the recording of patient symptoms and diagnoses. ICD-10 became effective on October 1, 2015, but is not widely utilized yet.

4—**B and C**: Each ICD-9 code must be linked to the appropriate CPT code, that is, the diagnosis must match or be relevant to the procedure performed.

References

CMS.gov. http://innovation.cms.gov/initiatives/bundled-payments. Published 2015. Accessed January 3, 2016

American Medical Association. http://www.ama-assn.org/ama/pub/physician-resources/solutions-managing-your-practice/coding-billing-insurance/cpt.page. Published 2015. Accessed January 3, 2016

Jensen PR. A refresher on medical necessity. Fam Pract Manag 2006;13(7):28–32

Hirsch JA, Leslie-Mazwi TM, Nicola GN, et al. Current procedural terminology; a primer. J Neurointerv Surg 2015;7(4):309–312

Press MJ, Rajkumar R, Conway PH. Medicare's new bundled payments: design, strategy, and evolution. JAMA 2016;315(2): 131–132

Question 5. A radiology residency program requires all of its residents to participate in basic financial and business skill courses to understand coding, reimbursement, and billing mechanisms in preparation to effectively function in healthcare delivery systems. This is an example of which of the Maintenance of Certification (MOC) Six Core Competencies?

A. Medical knowledge

B. Interpersonal and communication skills

C. Practice-based learning and improvement

D. Systems-based practice

E. Patient care

F. Professionalism

Answer:

D—Correct! Systems-based practice. This involves demonstrating awareness of and responsiveness to the larger system of healthcare and the ability to effectively call on system resources to provide optimal value care.

A—Incorrect: Medical knowledge. This involves applying biomedical, clinical, and cognitive sciences to patient care.

B—Incorrect: Interpersonal and communication skills. This involves effectively exchanging information and teaming with patients, their families, and other healthcare professionals.

C—Incorrect: Practice-based learning and improvement. This involves investigating and evaluating your patient care which includes appraising your methods, assimilating scientific evidence, and improving your own practice.

E—Incorrect: Patient care. This directly involves the patient and must be compassionate, appropriate, and effective for treating health problems and promoting health.

F—Incorrect: Professionalism. This involves the physician's commitment to carrying out professional responsibilities, adhering to ethical principles, and demonstrating sensitivity to diverse patient populations.

Reference

Kavic MS. Competency and the six core competencies. JSLS 2002;6(2):95–97

Questions 6 to 8: A 65-year-old woman with diabetes and hypertension with a prior history of severe renal insufficiency undergoes an abdominal computed tomography (CT) with contrast. She is given 100 mL of low-osmolality contrast media (LOCM) intravenously. Four hours earlier, she had also received 100 mL of contrast for a chest CT.

Question 6. Based on the information provided, which of the following confers the greatest risk of developing contrast-induced nephropathy (CIN) in this patient?

A. Hypertension

B. Severe renal insufficiency

C. Diabetes

D. Repeat contrast administration in less than 24 hours

E. None of the above

Answer:

B—Correct! By consensus, preexisting severe renal insufficiency is the most important risk factor for CIN.

Question 7. At what serum creatinine or eGFR level is the risk of CIN so great that iodinated contrast should never be administered?

A. 1.5 g/dL or above

B. 2.0 g/dL or above

C. Less than 60 mL/min/1.73 m^2 or above

D. There is no absolute level

Answer:

D—Correct! There is no agreed-upon threshold. Taken directly from *The American College of Radiology (ACR) Manual on Contrast Media* "There is no agreed upon threshold of serum creatinine elevation or eGFR declination beyond which the risk of CIN is considered so great that intravascular iodinated contrast medium should never be administered." However, the level with the most evidence is a cutoff eGFR of 30 mL/min/1.73 m^2. For each case, the patient benefit–risk must be weighed. Most practices use a cutoff point serum creatinine level of 2.0.

Question 8. Which patients should be screened with serum creatinine prior to contrast administration?

A. Age > 60

B. History of renal disease

C. History of diabetes

D. Receiving medical therapy for hypertension

E. All of the above

Answer:

E—Correct! Also per *The ACR Manual on Contrast Media*, it is suggested for each of these scenarios that a serum creatinine measurement be obtained prior to administration of contrast. Also included in this category are those patients taking metformin or metformin-containing drugs.

Reference

The ACR Manual on Contrast Media. V 10.2. 2016. http://www.acr.org/quality-safety/resources/contrast-manual. Accessed September 2, 2016.

Questions 9 to 12: Match the following with the organization that oversees and maintains each of these areas:

A. Maintenance of Certification (MOC)
B. National Patient Safety Goal (NPSG)
C. Current Procedural Terminology (CPT)
D. Dose Index Registry (DIR)

Question 9. American Medical Association (AMA)

Question 10. The Joint Commission (TJC)

Question 11. The American Board of Radiology (ABR)

Question 12. The American College of Radiology (ACR)

Answers:

9—**C**: The CPT codes are maintained by the AMA (through an editorial panel).

10—**B**: The NPSG program was established by TJC in 2002 to help healthcare organizations address patient safety issues.

11—**A**: The MOC is a means for the ABR to verify physician competence and help facilitate/document professional development.

12—**D**: DIR was developed by the ACR. CT scanner data (including computed tomography dose index [CTDI$_{vol}$] and dose length product [DLP]) are collected in a registry and then returned to participating facilities. Each site can then compare its own numbers with those of other similar facilities. This allows tracking of performance and potential adjustment of scanning parameters and protocols.

References

Madewell JE, Hattery RR, Thomas SR, et al. Maintenance of certification. J Am Coll Radiol 2005;2(1):22–32

Carrizales G, Clark KR. Implementing protocols to improve patient safety in the medical imaging department. Radiol Manage 2015;37(4):26–30, quiz 31–32

Wilson JM, Samei E. Implementation of the ACR dose index registry. J Am Coll Radiol 2015;12(3):312–313

Question 13. Shortly after a patient is placed on a magnetic resonance imaging (MRI) scanner, he becomes unresponsive to verbal or painful stimulation. The emergency response team is immediately contacted. What is the next *best* step in management of this patient?

A. Check for a pulse, check for breathing, and instruct the emergency response team to immediately enter the MRI scanner room and begin resuscitation efforts.
B. Immediately remove the patient from the MRI scanner room.
C. Make sure the equipment is powered off before beginning resuscitation.
D. Check for a pulse, check for breathing, and remove all metallic objects before allowing the emergency response team to enter the MRI scanner room.

Answer:

B—Correct! The MRI scanner is in MRI Zone IV which is under the direct supervision of MR personnel. If there is a medical emergency, immediately remove the patient from the MRI scanner room prior to further stabilization or initiating resuscitation efforts. The emergency response team should perform their duties *outside* of this MRI Zone IV.

A, C, D—Incorrect: First and foremost, the patient must be removed from the MRI scanner room.

References

Bushong SC, Clarke G. Magnetic Resonance Imaging: Physical and Biological Principles. 3rd ed. St. Louis, MO: Mosby, Inc.; 2003

Westbrook C. MRI at a Glance. West Sussex, UK: Blackwell Science; 2013

Question 14. Regarding electronic transmission of health information and the Health Insurance Portability and Accountability Act (HIPAA), which of the following is the most correct?

A. Does not apply to health plans

B. Applies to healthcare clearinghouses

C. Does not apply to healthcare providers

D. Applies only to healthcare providers

Answer:

B—Correct! Electronic transmission of health information applies to healthcare clearinghouses as well as health plans and healthcare providers. Per 45 CFR Part 160 Subpart A, these organizations may also have business associates that require the electronic transmission/disclosure of individually identifiable health information. A business associate may include the healthcare provider's employees as well as "partners" that provide a variety of services, including legal, actuarial, accounting, consulting, data aggregation, management, financial, or administration duties.

References

Andriole KP. Security of electronic medical information and patient privacy: what you need to know. J Am Coll Radiol 2014;11(12, Pt B):1212–1216

HIPAA Survival Guide. www.hipaasurvivalguide.com. Published 2016. Accessed February 27, 2016

Question 15. Regarding the ACR Practice Parameters and Technical Standards, which of the following is most accurate?

A. They are developed solely by an ACR committee and represented by radiology and radiation oncology physicians.

B. They are intended to represent legal standards of care or conduct.

C. They are based upon current literature, open forum commentary, and informal consensus. Expert opinion may also be included.

D. They are intended for strict adherence. Opposing independent medical judgment/decisions are almost never acknowledged.

Answer:

C—Correct! They are evidence- and consensus-based principles and technical parameters.

A—Incorrect: They may be jointly developed with other professional organizations (i.e., not always solely by the ACR).

B—Incorrect: They are not intended to represent legal standards of care or conduct.

D—Incorrect: On occasion, acknowledgement is made on when independent medical judgment/decisions are provided.

Reference

ACR Practice Guidelines and Technical Standards. http://www.acr.org/Quality-Safety/Standards-Guidelines. Published 2015. Accessed February 27, 2016

Question 16. An example of lossless compression is:
A. Graphics Interchange Format
B. Joint Photographic Experts Group
C. Discrete Cosine Transform
D. Fractals

Answer:

A—Correct! Graphics Interchange Format (GIF). This is a method to reduce the amount of data needed to record an image (image data compression method). This is a mathematical technique that utilizes a reduced number of bits to represent the original image for the purpose of decreasing storage requirements and increasing the speed of transmission of the image. It is called LOSSLESS as there is no loss of information (**Fig. 2.1**). The compression ratio is usually 3:1.

B, C, D—Incorrect: In contrast, these represent LOSSY compression where the bits are also reduced but by identifying and removing marginally important information; this is irreversible and has a compression usually of about 10:1. These are additional methods to provide image data compression and represent LOSSY compression rather than lossless compression (there *is* a LOSS of information).

You may notice that when submitting images for publication, they may ask for .gif or .tif format rather than .jpeg for this reason; that is, no loss of information.

References

Kabachinski J. TIFF, GIF, and PNG: get the picture? Biomed Instrum Technol 2007;41(4):297–300

Gillespy T III, Rowberg AH. Displaying radiologic images on personal computers: image storage and compression: Part 1. J Digit Imaging 1993;6(4):197–204

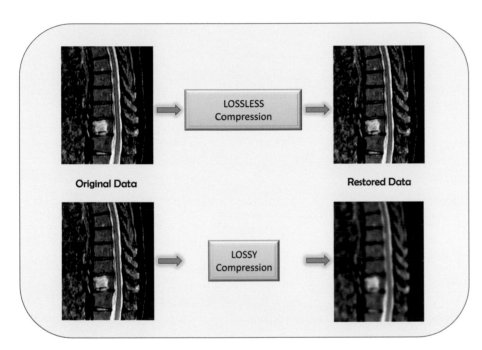

Fig. 2.1 Examples of LOSSLESS and LOSSY compression.

Question 17. Quality improvement (QI) may be differentiated from quality assurance (QA) by which of the following?
A. QI is more recent terminology.
B. QI only involves retrospective reviews.
C. QI attempts to avoid attributing blame.
D. A and C are correct.

Answer:

D—Correct! QI, the more recent terminology/concept of the two, is more of an umbrella term that includes QA. The ultimate "big picture" goal is to improve the care (performance and processes) delivered to patients by realizing organizational change. QI includes both retrospective and prospective reviews. QI also avoids blaming individuals.

B—Incorrect: QA includes only retrospective reviews and tends to identify adverse quality-related events.

References

Kruskal JB, Eisenberg R, Sosna J, Yam CS, Kruskal JD, Boiselle PM. Quality initiatives: Quality improvement in radiology: basic principles and tools required to achieve success. Radiographics 2011;31(6):1499–1509

Harvey HB, Hassanzadeh E, Aran S, Rosenthal DI, Thrall JH, Abujudeh HH. Key performance indicators in radiology: you can't manage what you can't measure. Curr Probl Diagn Radiol 2016;45(2):115–121

Questions 18 to 21: Match the following images with the appropriate flowchart (**Fig. 2.2**).

Question 18. Simple flowchart—A diagram that shows the sequential steps in a process from beginning to end.

Question 19. Spaghetti diagram—The route of an item or product as it travels down the value stream in an organization.

Question 20. Swim lane flowchart—The longitudinal visual representation of the sequence of events in an overall process or decision, with a lane for each person, group, or subprocess.

Question 21. Value stream map (VSM)—The entire map of a multidisciplinary process with visualization of its multiple data elements and the flow of information and material between them in order to deliver a product or service to the customer.

Answers:

18—**A**: *Various-shaped boxes* represent each sequential step or decision in a process. In other words, a simple flowchart shows an overall process and all of its associated steps. Examples of the different-shaped boxes and what they represent are as follows:

- Ovoid box—start or end of a process.
- Rectangular box—normal process flow step.
- Diamond-shaped box—a decision.
- Small circle—a connector.
- Parallelogram—data input or output.
- Box-shaped like a document—a document or report.

19—**D**: Each product is represented by a continuous line that traces its path as it travels in an organization. The route of the specific product looks like a spaghetti noodle.

20—**B**: *Parallel lines* give the chart the appearance of having swimming lanes and gives a longitudinal view of an entire process. The arrows represent how information or material is passed between subprocesses.

21—**C**: VSM provides visualization of an entire *multidisciplinary* process (all of its elements and flow of information and material between them) to demonstrate *supply to delivery to the customer*.

References

Singprasong R, Eldabi T. An integrated methodology for process improvement and delivery system visualization at a multidisciplinary cancer center. J Healthc Qual 2013;35(2): 24–32

Lean Six Sigma dictionary definitions: http://www.isixsigma.com/dictionary/spaghetti-diagram. Published 2016. Accessed February 27, 2016

Lee E, Grooms R, Mamidala S, Nagy P. Six easy steps on how to create a lean sigma value stream map for a multidisciplinary clinical operation. J Am Coll Radiol 2014;11(12, Pt A): 1144–1149

What do the different flowchart shapes mean: http://www.rff.com/flowchart_shapes.htm. Published 2016. Accessed February 27, 2016

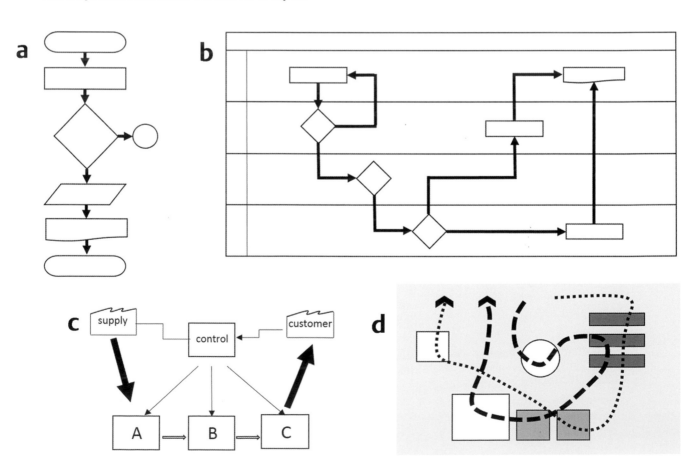

Fig. 2.2 Types of flowcharts.

Question 22. Which of the following best defines "value" in healthcare?

A.   The ratio of cost savings to cost of expended resources

B.   The cost-cutting measures utilized

C.   Health outcomes achieved per dollar spent

D.   Synonymous with relative value unit (RVU)

Answer:

C—Correct! Value should always be defined around the patient and their quality of care in the healthcare environment. It is measured by the outcomes achieved. Value also involves efficiency, since it pertains to outcomes relative to costs. Simply put, it is: OUTCOMES/COSTS, not income/costs or (cost savings)/expenses.

A and B—Incorrect: Value in healthcare is not solely related to monetary values.

D—Incorrect: RVU is a measure used to determine Medicare reimbursement for physician services.

References

Porter ME. What is value in healthcare? N Engl J Med 2010;363(26):2477–2481

McGinty G. Is value-driven healthcare an unfunded mandate for radiologists? AJR Am J Roentgenol 2016;206(2):280–282

Question 23. A newborn has been abducted from the hospital nursery. Which of the following best describes what has occurred?

A.   Code Pink alert

B.   Hospital security system failure

C.   Adverse event

D.   Sentinel event

Answer:

D—Correct! TJC set into place a Sentinel Event Policy in 1996. As defined by TJC, a sentinel event is "any unanticipated event in a healthcare setting resulting in death or serious physical or psychological injury to a patient not related to the natural course of the patient's illness." In other words, it is a patient safety event/unexpected occurrence that results in death, serious physical or psychological injury, or "the risk thereof." There must be an immediate investigation and response to a sentinel event.

A—Incorrect: Code Pink is a common term used in hospitals to alert that an infant is missing from the nursery. This is also a good answer choice but refers only to the *type of alert*.

B—Incorrect: This does not necessarily mean that the hospital security system has failed.

C—Incorrect: An adverse event is a more general term describing that an injury or undesirable clinical outcome has resulted *from medical care*.

References

http://www.jointcommission.org/assets/1/6/CAMH_24_SE_all_CURRENT.pdf. Published 2016. Accessed February 27, 2016

Jeffs L, Hayes C, Smith O, et al. The effect of an organizational network for patient safety on safety event reporting. Eval Health Prof 2014;37(3):366–378

JCAHO. What Every Hospital Should Know about Sentinel Events. 1st ed. Oakbrook Terrace, IL: JCAHO; 2000

Questions 24 to 27: The following questions refer to basic life support. Choose the *best* first step from the following list for each of the scenarios.

A. Activate an emergency response system.
B. Begin cardiopulmonary resuscitation (CPR) with chest compressions.
C. Begin rescue breathing.
D. Use the Heimlich maneuver.

Question 24. You are at a shopping mall and are the first to notice an elderly male on the floor. You have determined that he is unresponsive.

Question 25. You are at a park and see an unresponsive child on the ground. He is not breathing but does have a pulse. Someone else has already called 911.

Question 26. You are at your child's school gym. You are the first and only person on the scene when you determine that one of the children has experienced a sudden cardiac arrest.

Question 27. You are at a steak house enjoying a meal with your family when you notice that the lady at the next table is extremely distressed, clutching her neck, and making a high-pitched noise with each breath.

Answers:

24—**A**: In the Adult Chain of Survival, the next step is to activate the emergency response system and then begin early CPR with chest compressions. The five steps in the Adult Chain of Survival are as follows:

1) Immediate recognition of cardiac arrest and activation of the emergency response system
2) Early CPR with an emphasis on chest compressions

3) Rapid defibrillation
4) Effective advanced life support
5) Integrated postcardiac arrest care

25—**C**: For any age, when the victim has a pulse but is not breathing, begin with rescue breathing first. For adults, this means one breath every 5 seconds. For infants or children, this means one breath every 3 to 5 seconds. Give each breath over 1 second, and confirm that the chest is visibly rising.

26—**B**: In the Pediatric Chain of Survival, the next best step is to perform early high-quality CPR, then activate the emergency response system.

27—**D**: When you see someone choking, use the Heimlich maneuver for adults and for children age 1 year and over. For younger children/infants, use a combination of back slaps and chest thrusts, alternating them every five times.

References

Chain of Survival: http://www.heart.org/HEARTORG/CPRAndECC/WhatisCPR/EC%C2%ACCIntro/Chain-of-Survival_UCM_307516_Article.jsp#.VtKFLPkrKUk. Published 2016. Accessed February 27, 2016

Adult Rescue Breathing Training: http://www.procpr.org/en/training_video/adult-rescue-breathing. Published 2016. Accessed February 27, 2016

Berg MD, Schexnayer SM, Chameides L, et al. Part 13: Pediatric basic life support. 2010 American Heart Association guidelines for cardiopulmonary resuscitation and emergency cardiovascular care science. Circulation 2010;122:S862–S875

Epperly TD. Teaching the Heimlich maneuver. Postgrad Med 1990;88(8):31

Question 28. Regarding MRI safety zones, which is most accurate concerning the control room?

A. This is a Zone III area, under the supervision of MRI personnel, and with physical restrictions.
B. This is a Zone III area where access is unrestricted.
C. This is a Zone IV area, under the supervision of MRI personnel, and with physical restrictions.
D. This is a Zone IV area where access is unrestricted.

Answer:

A—Correct! Zone III is an area that must be supervised by MRI personnel and should have physical restrictions (such as locks).

B, C, D—Incorrect: The control room is considered an MRI safety Zone III, and access here has physical restrictions.

Reference

Tsai LL, Grant AK, Mortele KJ, Kung JW, Smith MP. A practical guide to MR imaging safety: what radiologists need to know. Radiographics 2015;35(6):1722–1737

Question 29. There are six Institute of Medicine (IOM) quality aims related to care. Select the one from the list below that is included among these six:
A. Serene
B. Equitable
C. Tenacious
D. Functional

Answer:
B—Correct! Equitable. This refers to providing patient care impartially and free from bias related to race, ethnicity, insurance status, income, or gender. The others are as follows:

1. Safety—To improve patient safety by reducing medical errors and adverse events.
2. Effectiveness—To incorporate the best research evidence, patient values, and clinical expertise for the purpose of providing the best patient outcomes.

3. Timeliness—To improve patient outcomes by the incorporation of timely and effective communication/intervention.
4. Patient-centered—To improve interactions between practitioners and their patients. This should encompass empathy, compassion, and respect for all patients.
5. Efficient—To deliver cost-effective and efficient healthcare to patients without compromising the quality of care.

A, C, D—Incorrect: These are not listed aims.

References
Slonim AD, Pollack MM. Integrating the Institute of Medicine's six quality aims into pediatric critical care: relevance and applications. Pediatr Crit Care Med 2005;6(3):264–269

Gamm L, Kash B, Bolin J. Organizational technologies for transforming care: measures and strategies for pursuit of IOM quality aims. J Ambul Care Manage 2007;30(4):291–301

Question 30. A patient is in the interventional radiology suite for a procedure. Which of the following is correct regarding identification of the patient prior to the procedure? Choose *all* that apply.
A. Two patient identifiers are required.
B. Patient identifiers may include Social Security number (SSN) last four digits, patient name, patient telephone number, patient identification number, or a government-issued ID.
C. Sources of patient identifiers include the patient, guardian, domestic partner, or a healthcare provider who has previously identified the patient.

Answer:
A, B, C. Correct! These are all correct. Patient identifiers include those listed in answer choice B above as well as the patient's date of birth and the last four digits of their SSN. Note that patient room number and/or location cannot be utilized as a patient identifier.

References
Reid-Paul TS. Radiologic Technology at a Glance. Clifton Park, NY: Delmar Cengage Learning; 2011

Cooper K, Gosnell K. Foundations and Adult Health Nursing. St. Louis, MO: Elsevier Mosby; 2015

For questions 31 through 34, match the description with the *best* choice of image (**Fig. 2.3**). The central portion of the target is assumed to be the true value:

Question 31. Precise and accurate.

Question 32. Accurate but not precise.

Question 33. Precise but not accurate.

Question 34. You have measured the Hounsfield units of an adrenal adenoma on CT five times. The measurements are exactly the same all five times, and all demonstrate an expected value to confirm an adrenal adenoma. Which image in **Fig. 2.3** best demonstrates your measurement results?

Answers:

31—**A**—Precise and accurate: near the same location each time, and therefore, reproducible. Accurate: close to the true value each time.

32—**D**—Accurate but not precise: close to the true value each time. Not precise: since each arrow is not close to each of the others, and therefore, not reproducible.

33—**B**—Precise but not accurate: near the same location each time, and therefore, reproducible. Not accurate: since none are close to the true value.

34—**A**—Precise: The measurements are precise since they are all close to each other. They are also accurate since they are all close to the expected value.

Of note, C is neither accurate nor precise.

References

Bourne R. Fundamentals of Digital Imaging in Medicine. Sydney, Australia: Springer-Verlag; 2010

Glaser AN. High-Yield Biostatistics. 3rd ed. Philadelphia, PA: Lippincott Williams & Wilkins; 2014

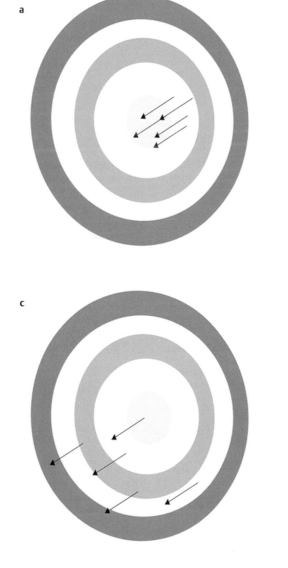
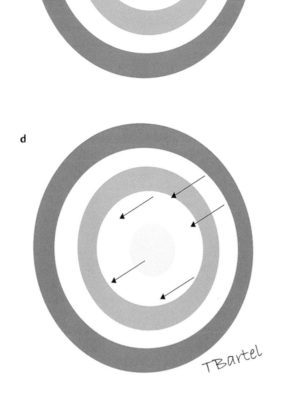

Fig. 2.3 Precision and accuracy.

Question 35. Which of the following refers to a phenomenon where adverse event reporting for a newly approved drug may increase during the first 2 years after its introduction?
A. Hawthorne effect
B. Observer effect
C. Weber effect
D. New drug effect

Answer:

C—Correct! Weber effect. This effect may occur after the introduction of a new agent or new indication for a drug. After 2 years, adverse effects subsequently start to decline. The Weber effect has been reported with gadolinium products and resultant allergic-like reactions among other medications. However, the Food and Drug Administration (FDA) conducted a large study in 2014 where this effect was not supported.

A, B—Incorrect: The Hawthorne effect (also called the Observer effect) explains that behavioral changes and productivity increases occur when workers are made aware that they are being observed. This is based upon research conducted in the 1920s in Illinois to determine which factors affected manufacturing productivity. A recent publication demonstrated this effect in radiology where real-time monitoring increased productivity.

D—Incorrect: The new drug effect is not an actual description of any effect.

References

Davenport MS, Dillman JR, Cohan RH, et al. Effect of abrupt substitution of gadobenate dimeglumine for gadopentetate dimeglumine on rate of allergic-like reactions. Radiology 2013; 266(3):773–782

Hoffman KB, Dimbil M, Erdman CB, Tatonetti NP, Overstreet BM. The weber effect and the united states food and drug administration's adverse event reporting system (FAERS): analysis of sixty-two drugs approved from 2006 to 2010. Drug Saf 2014;37(4):283–294

Kidwai AS, Abujudeh HH. Radiologist productivity increases with real-time monitoring: the Hawthorne effect. J Am Coll Radiol 2015;12(11):1151–1154

Questions 36 to 39. The following pertain to communication of image findings. For each scenario, select the best method of communicating the results.
A. Standard communication
B. Level 1 nonstandard communication
C. Level 2 nonstandard communication
D. Level 3 nonstandard communication

Question 36. You are reading a noncontrast CT of the head (of an elderly man who had fallen) and see an intracerebral hemorrhage.

Question 37. You are interpreting and dictating a screening mammogram and do not see any concerning findings.

Question 38. You are interpreting a positron emission tomography (PET)/CT in a patient with multiple myeloma. You note that there is focal fludeoxyglucose uptake in the right proximal femur which corresponds to an expansile lytic lesion with an extremely thinned cortex on the CT portion of the study.

Question 39. You are reading a noncontrast CT and detect a nonspecific solid adrenal nodule.

Answers:

Effective communication is an essential part of diagnostic imaging. It is important to be familiar with the levels of communication and their requirements.

36—B: This is considered a critical result and requires rapid and direct communication within 30 to 60 minutes of detection. Critical results mandate level 1 nonstandard communication, since these findings are new or unexpected and may be life-threatening or require an immediate change in patient management. Level 1 communication requires documentation of the interaction with the requesting clinician (or other licensed healthcare provider responsible for the patient's care). Documentation of level 1 communication may be audited.

37—A: This requires standard communication which refers to the creation and delivery of a written report (usually with an electronic format). The final report should ultimately reach the referring physician or healthcare worker that provides the patient's clinical follow-up.

38—C: In this case, the concern is for an impending fracture. This is classified as a level 2 nonstandard communication of results. A finding of this type could result in significant morbidity or even mortality. The results must be communicated within 6 to 12 hours and may be directly communicated either by a radiologist or by a designated associate on the radiologist's behalf.

39—D: This is classified as a level 3 nonstandard communication with non–time-sensitive results. Although this may involve a new or unexpected imaging finding, communication is not urgent.

References

ACR Practice Parameter for communication of Diagnostic Imaging Findings. Reston, VA: ACR; 2014

Berlin L. Communicating results of all outpatient radiologic examinations directly to patients: has the time come? AJR Am J Roentgenol 2009;192:571–573

Question 40. An extensive femoral vein thrombus is missed on CT. What type of error is this best classified as?

A. Perceptual error

B. System error

C. Preventive error

D. Communication error

Answer:

A—This is a perceptual error which is typically an error of scanning, recognition, or interpretation. This includes misses when interpreting images.

B—Incorrect: A system error is due to a context of delivery error or system issue and could include a communication error or failure to communicate a result.

C—Incorrect: A preventative error is a type of medical error where there is failure to provide prophylaxis or there is inadequate monitoring or follow-up of treatment.

D—Incorrect: This scenario cannot have involved a communication error if the abnormal finding was not seen to begin with, and therefore, it was not known that there was a finding to be communicated.

It is reported by Lee et al that the retrospective error rate for radiology imaging studies is about 30%, and real-time errors are about 3 to 5%. They also state that about 75% of all malpractice cases against radiologists are due to diagnostic errors. This can at least partially be attributed to the increased demands of reading faster and reading higher volumes.

Diagnostic errors by radiologists are generally due to detection error, interpretation error, failure to communicate results properly, or failure to suggest the appropriate follow-up test.

References

Lee CS, Nagy PG, Weaver SJ, Newman-Toker DE. Cognitive and system factors contributing to diagnostic errors in radiology. AJR Am J Roentgenol 2013;201(3):611–617

Taylor GA, Voss SD, Melvin PR, Graham DA. Diagnostic errors in pediatric radiology. Pediatr Radiol 2011;41(3):327–334

Pescarini L, Inches I. Systematic approach to human error in radiology. Radiol Med (Torino) 2006;111(2):252–267

Questions 41 to 44. These questions refer to the following receiver operating characteristic (ROC) curves (**Fig. 2.4**):

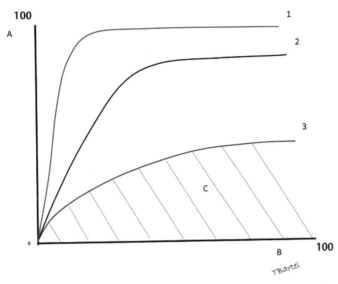

Fig. 2.4 Receiver operating characteristics (ROC) curves.

Question 41. What are the proper labels for A (*y*-axis) and B (*x*-axis)?
A. A: Specificity, B: Accuracy
B. A: 1−Specificity, B: Sensitivity
C. A: Sensitivity, B: 1−Specificity
D. D. A: 1−Sensitivity, B: Specificity

Answer:
C—Correct! The *y*-axis (A) represents sensitivity. This axis gives a range of true positives (TP) from low to high. The *x*-axis (B) represents 1-specificity (or 100%-specificity). This axis gives a range of false positives (FP) from low to high.

Question 42. Which curve represents the most ideal diagnostic test?
A. 1
B. 2
C. 3

Answer:
A—1—Correct! The ROC curve is a graphic plot demonstrating the performance of a binary classifier system. The TPs are plotted against the FPs at different thresholds or cut-off points, i.e., demonstrates the trade-offs between TPs and FPs across a series of cut-off points. This is useful in medicine in determining a cut-off point for a clinical test which ideally would have the highest sensitivity (highest *y*-axis value) and maximum specificity (smallest *x*-axis value). It is a good measure of test accuracy. In this case, this is best demonstrated by curve 1. An example would be determining the optimal cut-off value (highest sensitivity

and specificity) for a serum tumor marker to help differentiate between malignancy and nonmalignancy.

Question 43. What does C represent, and which numeric value represents a perfect test?
A. Area under the curve (AUC); 0.5
B. Area of consistency (AOC); 0.5
C. Area over the curve (AOC); 1
D. Area under the curve (AUC); 1

Answer:
D—Correct! This represents the AUC. The accuracy of a test is measured by the AUC of the ROC curve. An AUC of "1" is a perfect test, and an AUC of 0.5 is a failed test. The following are value guidelines for an AUC:

1−perfect
0.9 to 1−excellent
0.8 to 0 .9−good
0.7 to 0.8−fair
0.6 to 0.7−poor
0.5 to 0.6−fail

Question 44. ROC curve analysis does not depend upon _____.
A. Reader interpretation bias.
B. Defining a cut-off point.
C. Disease prevalence.
D. The relationship between sensitivity and specificity of a test.

Answer:
C—Correct! ROC curve analysis is independent of prevalence of disease, since it is based upon sensitivity and specificity.

A—Incorrect: Interpretation does depend upon the specific reader's interpretation bias (i.e., different decision thresholds) for classifying cases as normal or abnormal.

B—Incorrect: The curve is a continuum of cutoff points with the best cut-off point chosen for a particular diagnostic test.

D—Incorrect: Analysis does depend upon the relationship of sensitivity and specificity to determine the best cut-off point of a diagnostic test.

References
Bushberg JT, Seibert JA, Leidholdt EM, et al. The Essential Physics of Medical Imaging. 3rd ed. Philadelphia, PA: Lippincott Williams & Wilkins; 2012

Obuchowski NA. Receiver operating characteristic curves and their use in radiology. Radiology 2003;229(1):3–8

Lang TA, Secic M. How to Report Statistics in Medicine: Annotated Guidelines for Authors, Editors, and Reviewers. 2nd ed. Philadelphia, PA: ACP Press; 2006

Question 45. Which of the following are elements of informed consent for a proposed procedure? Choose *all* that apply.
A. Benefits
B. Reasonable alternatives
C. Every conceivable risk
D. Purpose of the procedure
E. All of the above

Answer:
A, B, D—Correct! The elements of informed consent for a procedure include discussing the benefits and potential risks as well as the reasonable alternatives to the procedure. The following are also required: purpose and nature of the procedure, method by which the procedure will be performed, possible complications, risks of declining the procedure, and the right to refuse the procedure. If these elements are lacking in the informed consent, a medical malpractice claim may be reinforced. Providing all of these elements creates a stronger informed consent, reduces potential physician liability, and increases the patient's role in making personal decisions.

References
ACR-SIR Practice Parameter on Informed Consent for Image-Guided Procedures. Reston, VA: ACR; 2014

Raab EL. The parameters of informed consent. Trans Am Ophthalmol Soc 2004;102:225–230, discussion 230–232

Cordasco K. Obtaining informed consent from patients: brief update review. In: Making Healthcare Safer II: An Updated Critical Analysis of the Evidence for Patient Safety Practices. Rockville, MD: Agency for Healthcare Research and Quality; 2013:461–471

Question 46. Regarding radiological peer review, all of the following are true *except:*
A. Data are protected from medico-legal discovery.
B. Data may be included in public reporting.
C. Data may be linked to Ongoing or Focused Professional Practice Evaluations (OPPE or FPPE).
D. RadPeer is an example of a radiology peer review program.

Answer:
B—Correct! Data should *not* be included in public reporting. Peer review is a quality *and* safety process in which peers randomly review other peers' work. This is often required by regulatory or accreditation bodies.

A—Incorrect: Data *are* protected from medico-legal discovery. In fact, there are federal and state laws that grant legal immunity from suits to those who participate in professional peer review (provided there is a genuine intention to help improve healthcare with the reviews).

C—Incorrect: Data *may* be linked to OPPE or FPPE.

D—Incorrect: RadPeer *is* one well-known radiological peer review system example which was created by the ACR.

Peer review is required by both ACR and TJC for accreditation.

References
Borgstede JP, Lewis RS, Bhargavan M, Sunshine JH. RADPEER quality assurance program: a multifacility study of interpretive disagreement rates. J Am Coll Radiol 2004;1(1):59–65

Mahgerefteh S, Kruskal JB, Yam CS, Blachar A, Sosna J. Peer review in diagnostic radiology: current state and a vision for the future. Radiographics 2009;29(5):1221–1231

Questions 47 to 50. Match the following scenarios with the appropriate MRI safety zones:

A—Zone I

B—Zone II

C—Zone III

D—Zone IV

Question 47. A patient and his wife are sitting in the waiting room/reception area.

Question 48. Location of the MRI scanner.

Question 49. A patient is putting on a hospital gown in a changing area.

Question 50. Location of the computer that controls the MRI scanner.

Answers:

(refer also to the associated image **Fig. 2.5**):

47—**A**—Zone I: This area is unrestricted to the public (i.e., open to the general public), and therefore, family members are permitted in this zone. Zone 1 is the entry area for the controlled MR environment. This is the only area that does not require MR personnel supervision.

48—**D**—Zone IV: This area is where the MRI scanner is housed and has the greatest potential for serious injury or death. It is under the direct supervision of MR personnel and the most tightly restricted (requiring the highest degree of supervision by MR personnel). Screened patients can be here if under MR personnel direct supervision.

49—**B**—Zone II: This is the least restrictive area of the zones which should be under supervision of MR personnel. This zone may house changing rooms or patient screening areas. This is where unscreened MRI patients would be located.

50—**C**—Zone III: This a more strictly controlled area under MR personnel supervision (as compared to Zone II). This includes the control room. Screened MRI patients can be in this area.

Tip: MRI-compatible permanent pacemakers should be set to the MRI safe mode while the patient is OUTSIDE of the MRI safety zones.

References

Raj V, O'Dwyer R, Pathmanathan R, Vaidhyanath R. MRI and cardiac pacing devices—beware the rules are changing. Br J Radiol 2011;84(1005):857–859

Gilk T. Working together to improve MRI safety. Jt Comm Perspect Patient Saf 2007;7:1–12

Kanal E, Barkovich AJ, Bell C, et al; Expert Panel on MR Safety. ACR guidance document on MR safe practices: 2013. J Magn Reson Imaging 2013;37(3):501–530

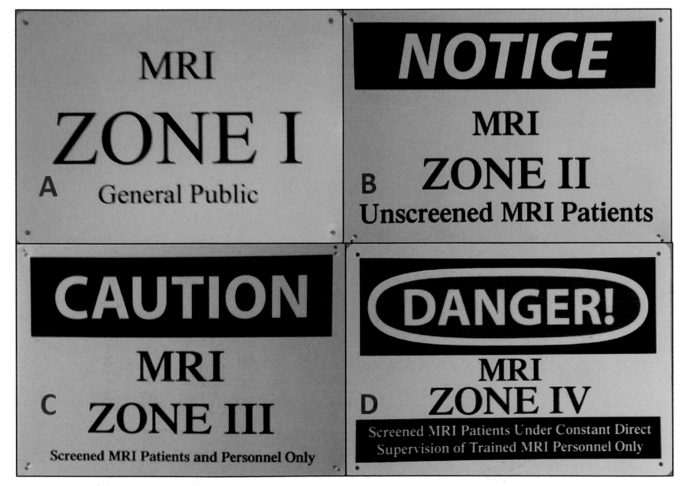

Fig. 2.5 MRI safety zone signs.

Question 51. Which of the following statements best describes the method of root cause analysis (RCA)?
A. The central tenet is to determine which individual(s) caused a healthcare mistake resulting in a serious adverse event.
B. The ultimate goal is to discipline the individual or individuals who caused the adverse event.
C. It involves establishing a protocol to analyze the sequence of events that led to an error/adverse event in order to prevent that event from recurring.
D. The goal is to identify active, not latent, errors.

Answer:

C—Correct! RCA is a structured protocol or method utilized in healthcare, within a culture of safety, to identify underlying problems that increase the likelihood of errors. The protocol may involve data collection, records review, and participant interviews which are then analyzed by a multidisciplinary team. RCA includes identifying both active and latent errors. TJC now requires that an RCA system be performed within 45 days for all sentinel and major adverse events.

A—Incorrect: The goal is to discover the underlying problem that led to a mistake for the purpose of future prevention (not simply to identify the "guilty" party).

B—Incorrect: The ultimate goal is to prevent future similar adverse events or errors by putting a preventative protocol into place.

D—Incorrect: RCA does not stop with simply identifying the active error. Latent errors are also sought out. In addition, a system to preventing future similar errors must be established.

References

Brook OR, Kruskal JB, Eisenberg RL, Larson DB. Root cause analysis: learning from adverse safety events. Radiographics 2015;35(6):1655–1667

Pinto A, Caranci F, Romano L, Carrafiello G, Fonio P, Brunese L. Learning from errors in radiology: a comprehensive review. Semin Ultrasound CT MR 2012;33(4):379–382

Choksi VR, Marn C, Piotrowski MM, Bell Y, Carlos R. Illustrating the root-cause-analysis process: creation of a safety net with a semiautomated process for the notification of critical findings in diagnostic imaging. J Am Coll Radiol 2005;2(9):768–776

Question 52. Which *best* describes a "standardized lexicon?"
A. It is a standardized set of terminology used to describe and classify findings.
B. It is similar to a medical dictionary but is a shorter version for radiological terms.
C. It has the same meaning as a "structured report."
D. It is only utilized in radiology.

Answer:

A—Correct! It helps to unify the language of radiology in reports. Some examples are the BIRADS for mammography, ultrasound, and MRI; LI-RADS for hepatocellular carcinoma; and Radiological Society of North America's (RSNA's) RadLex. It is argued that a standardized lexicon in radiology will improve patient care, outcomes, peer review, etc. However, there is also the potential of decreased productivity (and possibly accuracy) with what is termed an "eye-dwell" problem. This is where use of structured reports may cause an image interpreter to periodically take his or her eyes off the image while looking at the report templates.

B—Incorrect: It is not a collection of term definitions, but rather, a standardized vocabulary for a particular profession—in our case, for radiology.

C—Incorrect: However, note that standardized lexicons may comprise a component of a structured report; for example, standardized template for reporting, organizing, and formatting for the radiology institution.

D—Incorrect: Lexicons are not solely utilized in radiology (or even medicine).

References

Santillan CS, Tang A, Cruite I, Shah A, Sirlin CB. Understanding LI-RADS: a primer for practical use. Magn Reson Imaging Clin N Am 2014;22(3):337–352

Reiner BI, Knight N, Siegel EL. Radiology reporting, past, present, and future: the radiologist's perspective. J Am Coll Radiol 2007;4(5):313–319

RSNA. www.rsna.org/radlex.aspx. Published 2016. Accessed March 5, 2016

Hall FM. The radiology report of the future. Radiology 2009;251(2):313–316

Question 53. If the amount of spread around the mean of a data set is 16, the calculated standard deviation (SD) is:
A. 16
B. 32
C. 4
D. 8

Answer:
D—Correct! Variance and SD are utilized to measure the dispersion or spread of the data set around the mean, as opposed to central tendency, which measures the center of the data. (This is further discussed under mean, median, and mode in a separate question.) The SD is the square root of the variance. Therefore, the correct answer is 4.

One may think of SD as an index of variability. In general, a low SD means the data are less spread out, have less variability, and are more reliable. SD is always positive, because it is a distance.

References
Barde MP, Barde PJ. What to use to express the variability of data: Standard deviation or standard error of mean? Perspect Clin Res 2012;3(3):113–116

How to Find Variance and Standard Deviation: http://www.qa.dummies.com/education/math/statistics/how-to-find-the-mean-variance-and-standard-deviation-of-a-binomial-distribution/ Published 2016. Accessed September 7, 2016

Jackson HL. Mathematics of Radiology and Nuclear Medicine. St. Louis, MO: Warren Green, Inc; 1971

Sonnad SS. Describing data: statistical and graphical methods. Radiology 2002;225(3):622–628

Questions 54 to 57: Match the appropriate radiation exposure reduction initiative to the correct targeted population.
A. Image Gently
B. Image Wisely
C. Dose Index Registry (DIR)
D. Step Lightly

Question 54. Children

Question 55. Adults

Question 56. Interventional radiology and children

Question 57. All patients

Answers:
54—**A**: Image Gently was formed in 2006 by the Society of Pediatric Radiology and later named the Alliance for Radiation Safety in Pediatrics when other organizations joined in the initiative. The primary objective is to adjust radiation doses for the safe imaging of children. However, the ultimate goal is to change practices through improving staff and parent communications, reviewing protocols and implementing needed adjustments, and listening to suggestions from all imaging team members. The three phases used to disseminate this message include imaging professionals, referring physicians, and parents and the public.

55—**B**: Subsequently in 2009, a task force for adult radiation protection was jointly formed by the ACR and RSNA. The objectives and goals were similar to the Image Gently initiative but intended for adults. The primary focus was for CT imaging.

56—**D**: This campaign is primarily directed toward reducing pediatric radiation doses during pediatric interventional radiology. There are three key messages: (1) "Step lightly" on the fluoroscopy pedal, (2) "child-size" the protocol, and (3) consider alternative imaging such as ultrasound or MRI.

57—**C**: This was developed by the ACR. CTDIvol and DLP data from participating sites are sent to the DIR where it is then summarized and returned to allow comparison between the sites in order to track performance and adjust scanning parameters/protocols.

References
Image Gently: www.imagegently.org. Published 2014. Accessed March 5, 2016

Image Wisely: www.imagewisely.org. Published 2016. Accessed March 5, 2016

Interventional radiology: http://www.imagegently.org/Procedures/Interventional-Radiology. Published 2014. Accessed March 5, 2016

Sidhu M, Goske MJ, Connolly B, et al. Image Gently, Step Lightly: promoting radiation safety in pediatric interventional radiology. AJR Am J Roentgenol 2010;195(4):W299-301

Goske MJ, Applegate KE, Boylan J, et al. The 'Image Gently' campaign: increasing CT radiation dose awareness through a national education and awareness program. Pediatr Radiol 2008;38(3):265–269

Brink JA, Amis ES Jr. Image Wisely: a campaign to increase awareness about adult radiation protection. Radiology 2010;257(3):601–602

Questions 58 to 62. The following refer to this table and other related concepts (**Fig. 2.6**):

	(+) Disease	(-) Disease
(+) Test	80	5
(-) Test	20	95

Fig. 2.6 Test–disease contingency table.

A. 16
B. 83%
C. 8
D. 88%
E. Specificity

Question 58. Calculate the negative predictive value (NPV).

Question 59. Calculate the accuracy.

Question 60. Calculate the positive likelihood ratio (LRp).

Question 61. A test with high (choose: sensitivity or specificity) is most useful for ruling in a disease.

Question 62. The probability of disease in an exposed group is 40%. The probability of disease in an unexposed group is 5%. Calculate the relative risk (RR).

Answers:

58—**B**—83%. See the calculations in the table. This is the proportion of individuals with a negative test who do not have the disease. This answers the question: "If a test result is negative, how likely is it that the individual does not have the disease?" NPV is dependent upon disease prevalence.

59—**D**—88%. Accuracy = (TP + TN)/(TP + TN + FP + FN). For this case: (80 + 95)/(80 + 95 + 5 + 20) = 175/200. Accuracy is the sum of all true positives and negatives which is then divided by all cases. Comparing a measurement to a reference standard that is closest to the truth assesses accuracy. Accuracy depends upon disease prevalence.

60—**A**—16. LRp = Sensitivity/(1 − Specificity) = TP/FP. For this case: 80/5 = 16. This expresses how much more likely an individual with a positive test has the disease (TP), compared to someone with a negative test (FP). On the other hand, a negative likelihood ratio (LRn) is calculated by (1 − sensitivity)/specificity = FN/TN. There is convincing diagnostic evidence if LRp is >10 and LRn is <0.1, and strong diagnostic evidence if LRp is >5 and LRn is <0.2. Likelihood ratios help to assess the potential utility of a diagnostic test, and to assess how likely it is that an individual has the disease or condition. These are independent of disease prevalence.

61—**E**—Specificity. From the ABR noninterpretive skills study guide, "SPIN" is mentioned to remember **SP**ecificity to rule **IN**. In other words, a test with high specificity means that if the result is positive, there is a high chance of an individual actually having the disease. High specificity tests have low Type I error rates. (A Type I error is the case of rejecting the null hypothesis when it is in fact true.)

62—**C**—8. This is also sometimes called risk ratio and is commonly used in healthcare to calculate the risk of a specific population compared to the entire population. (Probability of disease in an exposed group)/(Probability of disease in an unexposed group) = 0.4/0.05 = 8. Therefore, we can say that the probability of disease in an unexposed group is eight times as likely as the probability of disease in the unexposed group (**Fig. 2.7**).

References

Riffenburgh RH. Statistics in Medicine. 3rd ed. San Diego, CA: Elsevier Inc.; 2012

Akobeng AK. Understanding diagnostic tests 1: sensitivity, specificity and predictive values. Acta Paediatr 2007;96(3): 338–341

Mayer D. Essential Evidence-Based Medicine. Cambridge: Cambridge University Press; 2004

	(+) Disease	(-) Disease	
(+) Test	80 (TP)	5 (FP)	PPV = TP/(TP+FP) = 94%
(-) Test	20 (FN)	95 (TN)	NPV = TN/(TN+FN) = 83%
	Sensitivity = TP/(TP+FN) = 80%	Specificity = TN/(TN+FP) = 95%	

Fig. 2.7 Test–disease contingency table with calculations.

Question 63. This is an alert system that signals readiness for additional parts or work.
A. Pull system
B. Kanban
C. LEAN system
D. Toyota Production System (TPS)

Answer:

B–Correct! Kanban. All of the choices above are interrelated in that they are all methods useful for optimizing operations. LEAN or lean process improvement has its roots in postwar Japan and is also related to the TPS continuous improvement practice, smoothness of workflow from end to end, and identification of waste as any element of workflow that does not add value to the end product or consumer. Along the lines of "not wasting" are the pull systems and Kanban. With a pull system, the next step of work only occurs immediately after the completion of a prior step. No single step creates more than the next can handle. This is where Kanban, a Japanese term, comes into play. Kanban is a just-in-time alert system that signals when the next step is ready for more parts or work. For example, this may involve a signboard or billboard.

References

Mitka E. Application of Kanban System on a hospital pharmacy. Hell J Nucl Med 2015;18(Suppl 1):4–10

Rawson JV, Kannan A, Furman M. Use of process improvement tools in radiology. Curr Probl Diagn Radiol 2016;45(2):94–100

Wormsley JM. A practical application of just-in-time. Hosp Mater Manage 1986;11(10):13–16

Question 64. Six Sigma targets a defect rate of _____ per million opportunities.
A. 3.4
B. 6.0
C. 6.6
D. 2.4

Answer:

A—Correct! 3.4 per million opportunities. Six Sigma was developed by Motorola and is a form of process improvement used to identify and remove the causes of defects (errors that occur during any process resulting in unexpected outcomes) and to minimize the variability in manufacturing and business. In total, 99.99966% of all opportunities to produce a part are statistically expected to be free of defects—that is, 3.4 defective features/million opportunities. Six Sigma is a methodology for eliminating defects aiming for six SDs between the mean and the nearest specification product.

References

Erturk SM, Ondategui-Parra S, Ros PR. Quality management in radiology: historical aspects and basic definitions. J Am Coll Radiol 2005;2(12):985–991

Benedetto AR. Six Sigma: not for the faint of heart. Radiol Manage 2003;25(2):40–53

Kubiak TM. Perusing process performance metrics: selecting the right measures for managing processes. Quality Progress; 2009. http://asq.org/quality-progress/2009/08/34-per-million/perusing-process-performance-metrics.html

---

Question 65. Which of the following may be inter-related? Choose *all* that apply.
A. Voice of the customer (VOC)
B. Key performance indicators (KPIs)
C. Dashboards
D. Flowcharts

Answer:

B and C—Correct! KPIs are selected measures to evaluate organizational goals. These may relate to financial measures, quality measures, customer service, or even appropriateness of image utilization. KPIs are commonly reported and displayed on organizational dashboards (visual representations of real-time key information). An example of a KPI specific to radiology would be instantaneous display on a computer-generated dashboard of an individual's image reporting turnaround time (TAT).

A—Incorrect: VOC is not related to dashboards or flowcharts, but rather, is a market research method used to identify customer wants which are then used to define new product definitions. This may take the form of a patient satisfaction survey. Therefore, VOC is more related to the customer, while KPI is more related to the organization.

D—Incorrect: A flowchart is not typically utilized to display KPIs. A flowchart is a diagram that visually demonstrates the sequential steps for a process or workflow.

References

Abujudeh HH, Kaewlai R, Asfaw BA, Thrall JH. Quality initiatives: key performance indicators for measuring and improving radiology department performance. Radiographics 2010;30(3):571–580

Karami M. A design protocol to develop radiology dashboards. Acta Inform Med 2014;22(5):341–346

Cull D. Process improvement: customer service. Radiol Manage 2015;37(5):53–56

Uberoi RS, Nayak Y, Sachdeva P, et al. Voice of the customer—a roadmap for service improvement. World Hosp Health Serv 2013;49(2):22–25

Questions 66 to 68: These questions pertain to the Medicare Payment Rate:

Question 66. Which of the following combinations is utilized in calculating the Medicare Payment Rate?
A. Specific Subspecialty Factor (SSF) + Relative Value Units (RVU) + Monetary Conversion Factor (CF)
B. RVU + Cost of Living Adjustment (COLA) + SSF
C. RVU + CF + GPCI
D. RVU + CF + GPC + SSF

Answer:
C—See **Fig. 2.8**. Note that RVU, GPCI, and CF are utilized in the Medicare Payment Rate Formula. COLA and SSF are not used in this formula. In fact, SSF is not existent and was created for this question. COLA stands for Cost of Living Adjustment and has been in effect since 1975 when it was initiated by the Social Security Administration as an automatic annual benefit increase to offset inflation.

Question 67. What is GPCI?
A. Gross Product Conversion Index
B. Geographic Practice Cost Index
C. Geographic Percentage Index
D. General Practicing Cost of Item

Answer:
B—GPCI stands for Geographic Practice Cost Index. This is used to help account for variations in the cost of practicing medicine in different parts of the country. RVU and GPCI are each multiplied by costs of malpractice insurance (MP), costs of maintaining a practice (PE), and cost of the physician's actual work. Each of these is then added up, and the total is multiplied by a dollar monetary conversion factor (CF) (**Fig. 2.8**).

RVU = Relative Value Unit. Three components.

PE RVU = Costs of maintaining a practice. This would include office space rental, cost of supplies and staffing.

MP RVU = Costs of malpractice insurance.

Work RVU = The actual work/service furnished. Accounts for about 50% of the total payment. See the next question for further information on this component.

GPCI = Geographic Practice Cost Index. Described above.

CF = Conversion Factor. Updated on an annual basis. It is equal to the Medicare Economic Index (MEI)—an inflation measure which is adjusted up or down per actual expenditures when compared to the target sustainable growth rate (SGR).

Question 68. The physician work component relative values are predominately based upon a Harvard study and include which of the following elements? Choose *all* that apply.
A. Technical skill and physical effort
B. Mental effort and judgment
C. Time required to perform the service
D. Cost of equipment to perform the service
E. Psychological stress of the physician (regarding iatrogenic risk to the patient)

Answer:
A, B, C, and **E** are all elements of the physician work component RVU. Congress authorized a 30-month study conducted by researchers at the Harvard School of Public Health in 1986. This was in conjunction with the AMA and was completed in 1988.

D—Incorrect: The cost of equipment needed to perform the service was not defined by the Harvard study as an element of physician work.

References

https://www.cms.gov/Outreach-and-Education/Medicare-Learning-Network-MLN/MLNProducts/downloads/Medcrephys-FeeSchedfctsht.pdf. Published 2014. Accessed on March 7, 2015

Kongstvedt PR. Essentials of Managed Healthcare. 6th ed. Burlington, MA: Jones and Bartlett Learning, LLC; 2013

Sidor G. Social Security: Cost-of-Living Adjustments. Washington, DC: Congressional Research Service; 2014:1–6

Glass KP. RVUs: Applications for Medical Practice Success. Englewood, CO: Medical Group Management Association; 2003

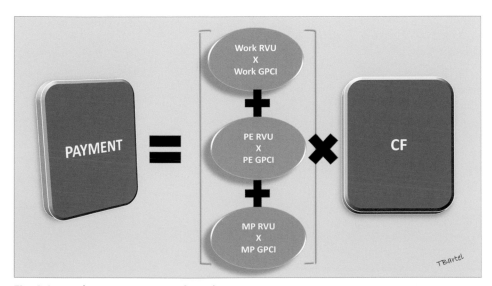

Fig. 2.8   Medicare Payment Rate formula.

Questions 69 to 73. Match the following scenarios with the type of factor that may lead to a latent error (also termed a latent condition).

A. Institutional/regulatory
B. Organizational/management
C. Work environment
D. Team environment
E. Staffing

Question 69. A nurse was asked to cover two additional shifts due to a mistake in scheduling. During the last shift (when she was exhausted), she mistakenly administered a morphine-containing product to a patient with a known morphine allergy. The patient subsequently had a severe allergic reaction.

Question 70. An interventional radiology division utilizes a large computer monitor in the preprocedure waiting area which identifies patients by last name and first initial only. A procedure was performed on the incorrect patient, and it was later discovered that there were two patients in the waiting area, both with the same last name and first initial.

Question 71. The surgery department is cutting costs, which includes purchasing less expensive latex gloves. These cheaper gloves have been used in the past, and the staff had complained that they ripped easily because of their lower quality. A surgeon is wearing these gloves during a procedure when the gloves rip, and the patient's blood comes into contact with an open wound on the physician's hand. The surgeon subsequently contracts HIV.

Question 72. A hospital modifies the flu shot policy, and now requires all employees to obtain this shot. A female employee taking anticoagulants subsequently develops a large hematoma after the shot, and this results in a prolonged hospitalization.

Question 73. An attending physician has started to perform a lumbar puncture on an inpatient. He is informed that the consent form has not been completed by the resident yet. The physician continues with the procedure.

Answers:

69—**E**: This is a problem with inadequate staffing. At first, this may seem like an active error, but the error is actually attributed to the system, which provided suboptimal staffing, leading to an exhausted and error-prone staff member.

70—**B**: Although this is a highly unlikely scenario, the example is an organizational/management issue. The preprocedure patient identification system is error prone.

71—**C**: This is a work environment error. Despite complaints of the poor quality of the gloves, the department was more concerned about cutting costs.

72—**A**: This is an institutional policy and regulation error. The rule was too stringent and discounted other potential consequences from the administration of this shot.

73—**D**: This case does not explicitly state that an active error was caused. However, this is considered a team environment error. In other words, the team member was not effective in safety/quality practice protocol. The attending physician was not displaying effective team collaboration or following protocol, nor was he portraying an effective team leadership model for the resident. This creates potential latent errors not foreseen yet.

These are all examples of latent errors which are typically unknown until an inciting event brings them to light. Latent errors occur at the blunt end and may be even more dangerous than active errors, since they are stealth and can result in multiple types of errors. Latent errors may be attributed to poor design, incorrect installation, poor management decisions, poor maintenance, etc., and, therefore, can be classified as institutional/regulatory, organizational/management, work environment, team environment, or staffing errors.

In contrast, an active error occurs at the sharp end at the point of contact between the provider and patient. These errors are discovered almost immediately.

Examples of active errors include pushing an incorrect button or ignoring some type of warning mechanism (when the equipment was entirely functional and installed correctly). An example of a latent error is faulty equipment installation when buttons were not installed in the correct locations or when the warning mechanism did not function.

References

Kattan MW. Encyclopedia of Medical Decision Making. Thousand Oaks, CA: Sage Publications; 2009

Carayon P, Wood KE. Patient safety - the role of human factors and systems engineering. Stud Health Technol Inform 2010;153:23–46

Moorman DW. Communication, teams, and medical mistakes. Ann Surg 2007;245(2):173–175

Question 74. A patient is undergoing a contrast CT study. Within seconds of contrast injection, the patient's blood pressure drops from 125/85 to 70/40, and the heart rate increases from 80 to 120 bpm. After routine basic treatment including elevating the legs, which of the following is the next *best* step in treatment?
A. Steroids
B. Labetalol
C. Epinephrine
D. Atropine

Answer:
C—Correct! This scenario represents an anaphylactoid reaction which typically includes both hypotension and tachycardia >100 bpm. If the hypotension persists after basic treatment (preserving IV access, monitoring vital signs, using pulse oximetry, elevating the legs, providing oxygen, and rapidly administering intravenous fluids), then the next recommended treatment is IV epinephrine 1 mL of 1:10,000 dilution (0.1 mg) slowly into a running infusion of IV saline. This can be repeated up to 1 mg total. EpiPen is an alternative.

A—Incorrect: Steroids are not indicated in this situation.

B—Incorrect: Labetalol is suggested for a hypertensive crisis, and atropine is suggested for bradycardia.

D—Incorrect: 0.6 to 1.0 mg of atropine may be given intravenously with a slow IV push for a severe vasovagal reaction (i.e., hypotension with bradycardia) followed by a saline flush. This can be repeated up to 3 mg total.

References
The ACR Manual on Contrast Media. V 10.2. 2016. http://www.acr.org/quality-safety/resources/contrast-manual. Accessed September 2, 2016

Pasternak JJ, Williamson EE. Clinical pharmacology, uses, and adverse reactions of iodinated contrast agents: a primer for the non-radiologist. Mayo Clin Proc 2012;87(4):390–402

Collins MS, Hunt CH, Hartman RP. Use of IV epinephrine for treatment of patients with contrast reactions: lessons learned from a 5-year experience. AJR Am J Roentgenol 2009;192(2):455–461

Question 75. Which of the following statements have some type of relationship to the BEIR VII Lifetime Risk Model? Choose *all* that apply.
A. This model predicts that about one person in 100 would be expected to develop solid cancer or leukemia from a dose of 100 mSv above background.
B. Sources for their studies included atomic bomb survivors.
C. They use a linear threshold model to estimate radiation risks.
D. They provide up-to-date information and risk estimates for cancer and other health effects from exposure to low-level ionizing radiation.

Answer:
A, B, D—Correct! All of these answer choices do have a relationship to BEIR VII. BEIR (Biologic Effects of Ionizing Radiation) VII is sponsored by federal agencies and provides comprehensive risk estimates for cancer and additional health-related effects from low-level ionizing radiation exposure. They use an linear NO-threshold (LNT) risk model, which demonstrates that at lower radiation doses, the risk of cancer does not have a threshold and proceeds in a linear fashion. In other words, there is no threshold below which there is no risk, and any low-LET ionizing radiation (levels up to 100 mSv) may increase the risk of cancer. There is a straight rising line in this model which means that health risk increases with increased exposure. BEIR VII heavily utilizes data from atomic bomb survivors in Japan and also uses data from individuals exposed at work in medical settings. With this, they statistically derive their conclusions.

C—Incorrect: They use an LNT model, not a linear threshold model, to estimate radiation risks.

References
Beir VII: health risks from exposure to low levels of ionizing radiation. *Report in Brief.* The National Academies Press. Washington, DC. http://dels.nas.edu/resources/static-assets/materials-based-on-reports/reports-in-brief/beir_vii_final.pdf. Accessed September 4, 2016

Davidson ST. Any dose is too high. Environ Health Perspect 2005;113(11):A735

This image is related to questions 76 and 77 below (**Fig. 2.9**).

Question 76. Regarding sources of radiation exposure in the United States, the blue semicircle above represents manmade sources, and the purple semicircle represents natural sources (about 50% for each category). Given this information, what is the likely radiation exposure contribution (percentage) from nuclear medicine?

A. 36%

B. 37%

C. 5%

D. 12%

Answer:

D—Correct! 12%. The largest source of manmade radiation exposure is from medical imaging and treatment (12 + 36 = 48%). Within medicine, the largest source of radiation exposure is from CT imaging which comprises about 24% of the 48%. The next most prevalent is nuclear medicine at about 12% and then interventional fluoroscopy at about 7%. On this chart, the 36% is the total from CT and interventional radiology (IR).

Question 77. Which organization collects and publishes data comparing ionizing radiation exposure to the U.S. population and its relative sources?

A. Nuclear Regulatory Commission (NRC)

B. American College of Radiology (ACR)

C. National Council on Radiation Protection and Measurements (NCRP)

D. Environmental Protection Agency (EPA)

Answer:

D—NCRP. The most recently published data are from 2009. From the early 1980s to 2006, there was a sixfold increase in total medical radiation exposure (15 to 48%). CT currently contributes the largest dose from medical imaging (**Fig. 2.10**).

(Of note, consumer products include tobacco products, smoke detectors, ceramics, and fertilizer, to name a few).

References

Schauer DA, Linton OW. NRCP Report No. 160: Ionizing radiation exposure of the population of the United States. Health Phys 2009;97(1):1–5

Health Physics Society. Fact sheet. 2015. www.hps.org. Accessed September 4, 2016

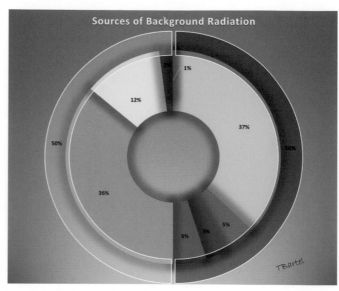

Fig. 2.9 Background radiation sources.

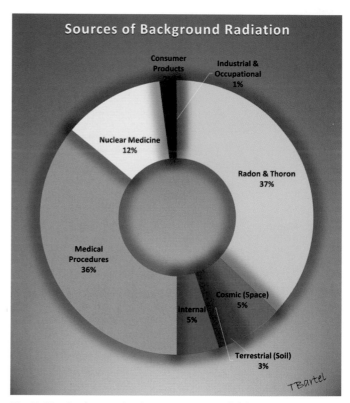

Fig. 2.10 Background radiation sources with labels.

Questions 78 to 80. Associate the provided description with the type of research study:

A. Cross-sectional

B. Case-control

C. Cohort

D. Experimental

E. Technology assessment

F. Meta-analysis

Question 78. Studies have already been published, and a systematic review of these studies is made to identify the relevant articles on a certain topic.

Question 79. All measurements are made at one point in time and can yield prevalence.

Question 80. An intervention occurs, and the effect on outcome is evaluated.

Answers:

78—**F**: Meta-analysis. These are high-level evidence. A statistical methodology is applied to the various results as if a single large study.

79—**A**: Cross-sectional. This is a prevalence study which describes variables and their distribution patterns, is fast and inexpensive, but is weak in establishing causation.

80—**D**: Experimental. This is also called a randomized controlled trial and is used in clinical trials. An advantage is that the cause of an effect from an intervention can be established. This is the most well-planned type of study providing the greatest degree of sound evidence.

Cohort study: Subjects are followed over time prospectively or retrospectively (follow-up study). Two healthy groups are followed over time. One group is exposed to something specific, while the other is not. These types of study can detect a cause between exposure of the specific substance and development of disease.

Case-control study: This type of study is retrospective and includes two groups, those who already have a disease (cases) and those without (controls). This type of study involves taking a look back in time (retrospective) to identify factors that might have been associated with the illness.

Technology assessment: This type of study is utilized when assessing any medical *technology* in healthcare.

References

Röhrig B, du Prel JB, Wachtlin D, et al. Types of study in medical research: part 3 of a series on evaluation of scientific publications. Dtsch Arztebl Int 2009;106(15):262–268

Cronin P, Rawson JV. Review of research reporting guidelines for radiology researchers. Acad Radiol 2016;23(5):537–558

Mayer D. Essential Evidence-Based Medicine. New York, NY: Cambridge University Press; 2004

Questions 81 and 82. Regarding the PDSA cycle (**Fig. 2.11**).

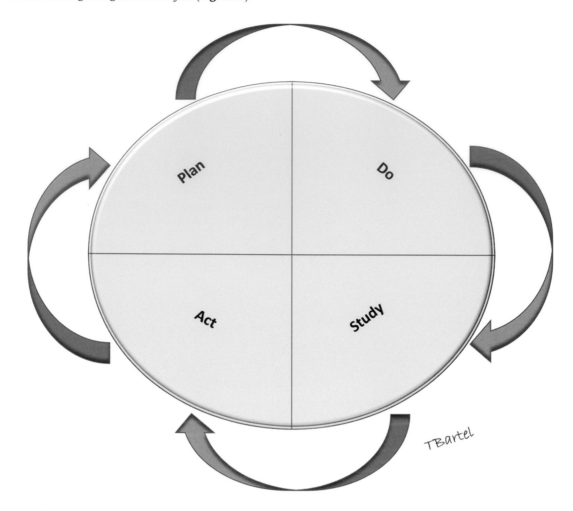

Fig. 2.11   The PDSA cycle.

A. Plan

B. Do

C. Act

D. Study

Question 81. Which step involves determining how well your measurements compare to the desired goal?

Question 82. Which step involves devising and implementing a means for performance improvement that addresses a perceived root cause of not achieving a target?

Answers:

81—**D**: Study—Determine how well your measurements compare to a desired goal, explore root causes for not achieving this goal, analyze baseline data to compare to the result, and summarize the results and what you have learned.

82—**C**: Act—Devise and implement performance improvement techniques to address the root cause. Do this before you re-measure.

Fig. 2.11 is a graphic demonstration of the PDSA cycle (or Plan–Do–Study–Act cycle). This is a four-step process that can be used for process improvement/continuous quality improvement (CQI). In fact, the cycle can be repeated several times, if needed, until the desired goal is reached. In addition to the descriptions above for Study and Act, the following are brief summaries of the Plan and Do steps:

- Plan—Identify an area that needs improvement and plan a way to measure it with a target goal. Devise a way to collect the measured data.

- Do—This is where your plan is put into action, make the baseline measurements, and collect the data.

References

Taylor MJ, McNicholas C, Nicolay C, et al. Systemic review of the application of the plan-do-study-act method to improve quality in healthcare. BMJ Qual Saf 2014;23(4):290–298

Tamm EP, Szklaruk J, Puthooran L, et al. Quality initiatives: planning, setting up, and carrying out radiology process improvement projects. Radiographics 2012;32(5):1529–1542

Rawson JV, Kannan A, Furman M. Use of process improvement tools in radiology. Curr Probl Diagn Radiol 2016;45(2):94–100

Questions 83 and 84. The following are related to gadolinium administration and nephrogenic systemic fibrosis (NSF):

Question 83. In which setting is there a greater-than-average risk for developing NSF? Choose *all* that apply.
A. eGFR ≥ 40
B. Acute renal injury or chronic renal disease
C. Patient on dialysis

Answer:

B and C—Correct! There is general consensus that exposure to gadolinium contrast in the setting of acute kidney injury or severe chronic renal disease is needed for NSF to develop. A patient on dialysis may be included in either of these categories.

A—Incorrect: There are no special precautions when the eGFR is ≥ 40.

Question 84. Which gadolinium contrast agent has the highest risk for NSF?
A. Gadodiamide (Omniscan)
B. Gadoteridol (ProHance)
C. Gadopentetate (Magnevist)
D. Gadoxetate (Eovist)

Answer:

A—Correct! Omniscan has a linear non-ionic structure and is more likely to release Gd (III). It is reported that 78% of cases are due to Omniscan. The least likely in this list to have resultant NSF is ProHance, as this is the least likely to release Gd (III) and has a macrocyclic structure. Magnevist and Eovist have an intermediate risk (and an ionic linear structure).

This clinical entity (NSF) was established in 2000. This is a scleroderma-like debilitating disease that occurs in patients with severe or end-stage renal disease linked to gadolinium administration. The patients develop erythematous skin plaques and eventually flexure contractures. Pathology presents weeks to months after the gadolinium administration. Organs besides the skin may also become involved. Precautions to preventing NSF should be taken in patients through appropriate screening prior to gadolinium administration. At-risk patients include solitary kidney, transplant kidney, renal neoplasm, age over 60 years, diabetes, and hypertension. The mechanism is suspected to be the dissociation of the gadolinium ion from its chelate which can then bind with an anion-like phosphate and subsequently deposit into tissues causing a fibrotic reaction. Of note, a macrocyclic structure means that a cage like ligand surrounds and tightly binds the Gd ion making these agents much more stable than those with linear structures. FDA-approved macrocyclic agents are gadoterate meglumine (Dotarem), gadobutrol (Gadavist), and gadoteridol (ProHance).

References

The ACR Manual on Contrast Media. V 10.2. 2016. http://www.acr.org/quality-safety/resources/contrast-manual. Accessed September 2, 2016

Idée JM, Fretellier N, Robic C, Corot C. The role of gadolinium chelates in the mechanism of nephrogenic systemic fibrosis: A critical update. Crit Rev Toxicol 2014;44(10):895–913

Perazella MA. Current status of gadolinium toxicity in patients with kidney disease. Clin J Am Soc Nephrol 2009;4(2):461–469

Kanal E, Maravilla K, Rowley HA. Gadolinium contrast agents for CNS imaging: current concepts and clinical evidence. AJNR Am J Neuroradiol 2014;35(12):2215–2226

Question 85. What is the most important takeaway point to recognize from the human reliability curve (**Fig. 2.12**)?

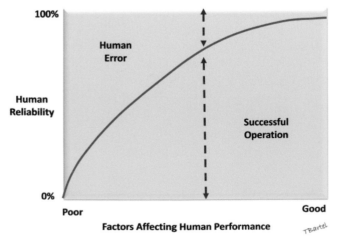

Fig. 2.12 Human reliability curve.

A. Many tasks are capable of 100% reliability.
B. No task will ever have 100% reliability.
C. As factors affecting human performance improve, reliability decreases.
D. As human error increases, human performance increases.

Answer:

B—Correct! The human reliability curve is a conceptual model for the management of human error showing the relationship between system design and the rate of human error. While human reliability improves with improvement in the factors affecting human performance, the curve never reaches 100%.

A—Incorrect: No task reaches 100% reliability.

C—Incorrect: Reliability increases as factors affecting human performance improve.

D—Incorrect: Human performance decreases with an increase in human error.

References

Abujudah HH, Bruno MA, eds. Quality and Safety in Radiology. New York, NY: Oxford University Press; 2012

Duffey RB, Saull JW. Managing and predicting technological risk and human reliability: a new learning curve theory, Part O. Journal of Risk and Reliability 2008;222(2):245–254

Question 86. Which of the following *best* describes LEAN? Choose *all* that apply.

A. Also known as the TPS

B. Represents an organizational style of CQI

C. Emphasis is on end-to-end smoothness of workflow

D. Relies on company culture

Answer:

A, B, C, D—Correct! The LEAN management style emerged around 1918 from postwar Japan. Subsequently, a book entitled *The Machine That Changed the World* (written in 1990) coined the word "lean." This style has a fundamental reliance on company culture and the following core management principles:

- Elimination of waste.
- Respect for long-term work relationships with mutual trust.

References

Teich ST, Faddoul FF. Lean management-the journey from Toyota to healthcare. Rambam Maimonides Med J 2013;4(2):e0007

Womack JP, Jones DT, Roods D. The Machine that Changed the World. New York, NY: Rawson Associates Scribner; 1990

Hutterer R. Toyota's Way of Production – Lean Production. Munich, Germany: GRIN Verlag; 2007

Liker JK, Convis GL. The Toyota Way to Lean Leadership. New York, NY: McGraw Hill; 2011

Question 87. A radiology imaging ordering system prompts the ordering physician either to verify a recent eGFR or to order one before a contrast CT can be requested. This is an example of:

A. Standardization

B. Resiliency effort

C. Forcing function

D. Work-around

E. Usability testing

Answer:

C—Forcing function. All of the techniques listed above are tools that can be used to address safety issues and human factors. This particular scenario is an example of a forcing function which can potentially prevent an unintended or undesirable action from occurring by first requiring a specific step to be performed (before the desired action is permitted). In this case, evaluation of renal function is required before the contrast CT can even be ordered.

A—Incorrect: Standardization. Standardizing equipment and processes helps to increase reliability, improve flow, minimize training needs, and ensure safety. This may utilize checklists.

B—Incorrect: Resiliency effort. This is a critical system property which is an aspect of risk management when an organization can anticipate and adapt to changing conditions.

D—Incorrect: Work-around. A work-around typically arises in situations when there are flawed or poorly designed systems. In those instances, a frontline worker bypasses a policy or safety procedure in order to complete a task more efficiently.

E—Incorrect: Usability testing. This is a process where human factor engineers test equipment or a process under a real-life scenario.

Human factors engineering (HFE) entails taking into account the fact that humans will make errors, and therefore, the systems with which humans will interact should be specifically designed to minimize those errors. HFE includes forcing functions, checklists, and processes standardization. Resiliency effort or engineering and usability testing also involve HFE, but are more of an organizational dynamic approach to risk management, rather than a specific technique like a forcing function. A work-around may occur when a process or task does not have a good human factors design, and therefore, the worker finds a way around the process to be more efficient and/or to complete the task. A work-around may increase risk to the patient.

References

Siewert B, Hochman MG. Improving safety through human factors engineering. Radiographics 2015;35(6):1694–1705

Larson DB, Kruskal JB, Krecke KN, Donnelly LF. Key concepts of patient safety in radiology. Radiographics 2015;35(6):1677–1693

Gluyas H, Morrison P. Patient Safety: An Essential Guide. New York, NY: Palgrave Macmillan; 2013

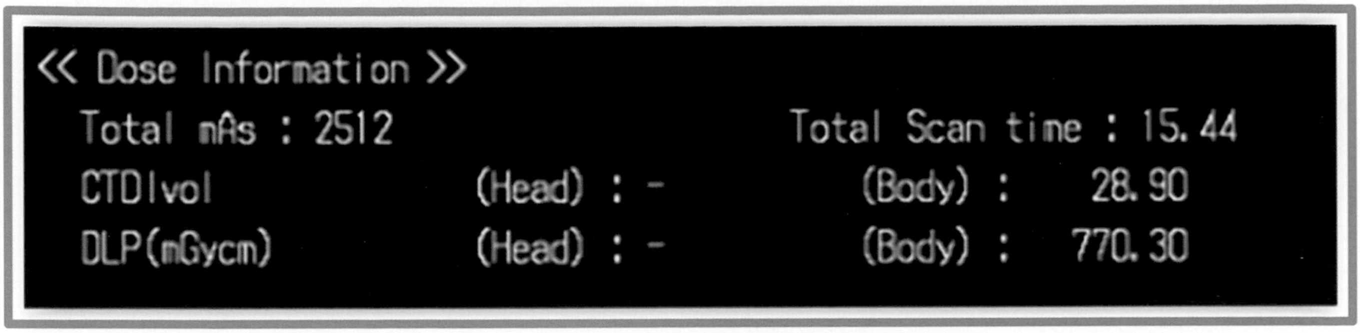

```
<< Dose Information >>
  Total mAs : 2512                  Total Scan time : 15.44
  CTDIvol              (Head) : -      (Body) :    28.90
  DLP(mGycm)           (Head) : -      (Body) :   770.30
```

Fig. 2.13 CT scan dose information.

Questions 88 and 89. Typical dose information is shown (see **Fig. 2.13**) for any particular CT scan.

Question 88. What is the unit of measurement for CTDIvol?
A. Milligray
B. Sievert
C. Milligray-cm

Answer:
A—Milligray (mGy).

B—Incorrect: Sievert (Sv) is an SI-derived unit of ionizing radiation, takes into account the type of radiation, and is used in calculating equivalent or effective dose. Gray is a measurement of the physical quantity of absorbed dose.

C—Incorrect: Milligray-cm (mGy-cm) is the unit for DLP which is (CTDIvol) (scan length) or (mGy) (cm).

Question 89. Determine the scan length with the information given.
A. ~ 77 cm
B. ~ 27 cm
C. ~ 50 cm
D. ~ 20 cm

Answer:
B—DLP (in mGy-cm) is the product of CTDIvol (in mGy) and scan length (in cm). Therefore, the correct answer is approximately 27 cm (770.30/28.90).

In a review performed by Huda et al, it was stated that CTDIvol and DLP are the only CT dose parameters that can be universally interpreted. CTDI is the radiation dose from a single CT slice. CTDI100 is the dose from a 100-mm range centered on the index slice. CTDIw (CTDI weighted) is the sum of two-thirds of the peripheral dose plus one-third of the central dose. CTDIvol is the CTDIw divided by the beam pitch factor. DLP is (CTDIvol)(scan length) where scan length is (slice thickness) (# of slices). One advantage of DLP is that it allows comparison between institutions for amounts of radiation utilized for similar examinations. Another advantage is that DLP can be converted into estimated dose to the patient.

References
Huda W, Mettler FA. Volume CT dose index and dose-length product displayed during CT: what good are they? Radiology 2011;258(1):236–242

Coursey CA, Frush DP. CT and radiation: what radiologists should know. Appl Radiol 2008;37(3):22–29

Question 90. Which is the *best* sequence and proper description of the Universal Protocol?
A. Mark the procedure site, conduct a procedure verification process, and perform time-out before the procedure.
B. Perform time-out before the procedure, mark the procedure site, and conduct a procedure verification process
C. Conduct a procedure verification process, mark the procedure site, and perform time-out before the procedure
D. Conduct a procedure verification process, perform time-out before the procedure, and mark the procedure site

Answer:
C—**Correct!** The Universal Protocol was enacted by TJC in 2004 and is a three-part process. (1) Conduct a preprocedure verification process, which includes verifying the correct procedure, patient, and site, as well as using a standardized list to verify items needed for the procedure. (2) The procedure site must be marked by the licensed practitioner responsible for the procedure (in some circumstances, by medical residents, physical assistants (PAs), etc.

(3) Perform a time-out immediately before the invasive procedure, which should include, at a minimum, correct identification of the patient, site, and procedure to be performed.

References
Angle JF, Nemcek AA Jr, Cohen AM, et al; SIR Standards Division; Joint Commission Universal Protocol for Preventing Wrong Site, Wrong Procedure, Wrong Person Surgery. Quality improvement guidelines for preventing wrong site, wrong procedure, and wrong person errors: application of the joint commission "Universal Protocol for Preventing Wrong Site, Wrong Procedure, Wrong Person Surgery" to the practice of interventional radiology. J Vasc Interv Radiol 2008;19(8):1145–1151

Ross J, Wolf D, Reece K. Highly reliable procedural teams: the journey to spread the universal protocol in diagnostic imaging. Perm J 2014;18(1):33–37

Mallett R, Conroy M, Saslaw LZ, Moffatt-Bruce S. Preventing wrong site, procedure, and patient events using a common cause analysis. Am J Med Qual 2012;27(1):21–29

Question 91. You are the interpreting radiologist for **Fig. 2.14.** What type of communication is required?

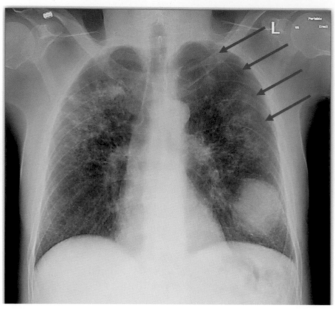

Fig. 2.14 Chest X-ray.

A. Level 1
B. Level 2
C. Level 3

Answer:

A—Correct! Level 1 results are considered critical when there are new or unexpected findings that are life-threatening or require an immediate change in patient management. There must be immediate and live communication to the ordering physician, a covering physician, or another care team member. Pneumothorax, as in this image, is one example. Other examples include acute deep vein thrombosis (DVT), acute intracerebral hemorrhage, ruptured aortic aneurysm, and unstable spine fracture.

B—Incorrect: Level 2 results are urgent but not critical and require communication within 6 to 12 hours. Communication can be live or a form approved by the institution. Examples include impending fracture and new or unexpected intra-abdominal processes.

C—Incorrect: Level 3 are not particularly time sensitive and typically conveyed in the electronic report. Examples include lung nodules and renal mass.

Of note, in contrast to Critical Results, a Critical Test is a TYPE of examination that requires rapid communication no matter what the finding is. An example is a CT PE protocol.

References

ACR. ACR Practice Parameter for Communication of Diagnostic Imaging Findings. Reston, VA: ACR; 2014

Berlin L. Communicating results of all radiologic examinations directly to patients: has the time come? AJR Am J Roentgenol 2007;189(6):1275–1282

Question 92. A nurse administers the wrong medication to an inpatient who then suffers a severe allergic reaction. Which of the following factors would classify this as an error on the sharp end?
A. This occurred despite having an appropriate identification and verification system in place for patient medications. However, the nurse did not utilize this process.
B. The medication labels were ambiguous, and there was no double check system in place.
C. The patient's record was missing allergy information.
D. The handwritten physician orders were difficult to read. The institution did not have a computer entry system in place.

Answer:

A—This is an example of an error at the sharp end (which occurs at the *front line)* involving the nurse's direct contact with the patient and her decision to proceed with administering the medication.

She knew that she did not verify the appropriate medication. This is also called an active error or active failure.

B, C, D—Incorrect: The other choices are examples of blunt errors (also called latent errors) which are due to *failures of organization or* design that affect the decisions of the person on the frontline.

References

Leroy P. Medical errors: the importance of the bullet's blunt end. Eur J Pediatr 2011;170(2):251–252

Brook OR, O'Connell AM, Thornton E, Eisenberg RL, Mendiratta-Lala M, Kruskal JB. Quality initiatives: anatomy and pathophysiology of errors occurring in clinical radiology practice. Radiographics 2010;30(5):1401–1410

Kohn LT, Corrigan JM, Donaldson MS. To Err Is Human: Building a Safer Health System. Washington, DC: National Academy Press; 2000

Questions 93 to 95. Match the following chart types with their descriptions.
A. **Fig. 2.15**
B. **Fig. 2.16**
C. **Fig. 2.17**

Question 93. Control chart

Question 94. Pareto chart

Question 95. Ishikawa diagram

Answers:

93–**C**: Control chart. This type of chart, also called Statistical Process Control, is used to analyze the performance of a system as a function of time. This visually displays the mean, median, upper, and lower control limits to help identify common causes (process noise), and special causes (those with significant deviation requiring attention). On this chart, the red dashed lines represent the upper and lower control limits. The lighter blue central area is due to normal variation (common causes). The data point 0.07 is an out-of-control point (special cause).

94–**A**: Pareto chart. Visually displays rank orderings of quality, safety, or risk factors by impact or importance. This chart is based upon the Pareto principle that states that a small number of steps contribute to the majority of the problems. The left-sided vertical axis is the frequency (# of counts for each category). The right-sided vertical axis is the cumulative percentage. The horizontal axis includes the group names of the response categories. Columns are arranged in descending order, and a cumulative line is also displayed to track percentages of each category or bar. This helps to visually demonstrate which categories have the greatest potential impact on problems or defects.

95–**B**: Ishikawa diagram. Used in RCA to identify all factors contributing to a problem. This is also called a Fishbone or Cause-and-Effect Diagram. This helps to visually display causes of an outcome and identify improvement opportunities.

References

Joiner Associates, Inc. Pareto Charts: Plain and Simple. Madison, WI: Joiner Associates, Inc.; 1995

Arthur J. Control charts for services. Quality Digest 2012. http://www.qualitydigest.com/inside/quality-insider-article/control-charts-services.html. Accessed September 4, 2016

Lighter DE, Fair DC. Principles and methods of quality management in healthcare. Gaithersburg, MD: Jones & Bartlett Learning, Aspen Publishers; 2000

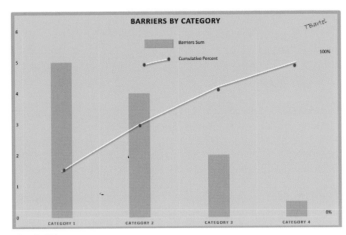

Fig. 2.15

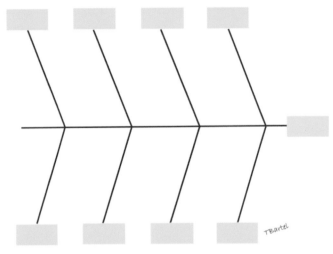

Fig. 2.16

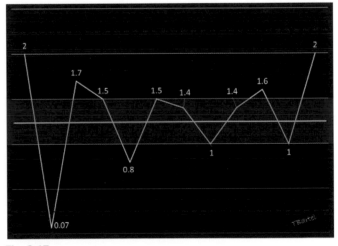

Fig. 2.17

Questions 96 to 98. Match the following scenarios with the type of error as published by the Institute of Medicine (IOM).
A. Diagnostic error
B. Treatment error
C. Preventative error

Question 96. A medication was ordered as an intramuscular (IM) administration but was given intravenously (IV) instead.

Question 97. A CT study was ordered with contrast, but for some unknown reason, contrast was not given.

Question 98. An I-123-MIBG scan was performed in a patient, but Lugol's solution was not prescribed beforehand per protocol.

Answers:
96–**B**: Treatment error. This particular example demonstrates one type of treatment error; that is, an error in how the treatment was administered to the patient. Other types of treatment errors include an error in the performance of an operation, procedure, or test, incorrect dose or method of using a drug, error in administering treatment, an avoidable delay in response to an abnormal test or delay in treatment, or care that is given but is not indicated.

97–**A**: Diagnostic error. In this example, a diagnostic imaging study was not employed in the manner that it was requested (with contrast). Other types of diagnostic errors include utilizing outdated tests or therapies, an error or delay in making a diagnosis, failure to employ the indicated test, or failure to act on the results of a test.

98–**C**: Preventative error. Lugol's solution is used as a preventative measure to reduce radioactive iodine uptake by the thyroid gland. Not administering this prior to the radiotracer injection, per protocol, represents a failure to provide prophylactic treatment. Inadequate monitoring or failure to follow up with a patient after treatment represents another type of preventative error.

References
Kohn LT, Corrigan JM, Donaldson MS. To err is human: building a safer health system. Washington, DC: National Academy Press; 1999

La Pietra L, Calligaris L, Molendini L, Quattrin R, Brusaferro S. Medical errors and clinical risk management: state of the art. Acta Otorhinolaryngol Ital 2005;25(6):339–346

Questions 99 to 101. Match the established ACR diagnostic CTDIvol reference value for each of the following:
A. 20 mGy
B. 25 mGy
C. 50 mGy
D. 75 mGy

Question 99. CT of the head—adult

Question 100. CT abdomen—5-year-old child

Question 101. CT of abdomen—adult

Answers:
These data are based upon the ACR CT Accreditation Program and allow facilities to compare their values to these reference values and make adjustments in scanning parameters when necessary.

In addition, each CT unit must pass both the clinical and phantom image quality test to obtain ACR accreditation. If the dose from the CT unit does not meet these criteria, the facility must repeat the entire portion of the phantom testing.

99–**D**—75 mGy—CT of the head of adult

100–**A**—20 mGy—CT abdomen of child

101–**B**—25 mGy—CT abdomen of adult

References

ACR. ACR CT Accreditation Program Requirements. Reston, VA: ACR; 2015

Mayo-Smith WW, Hara AK, Mahesh M, Sahani DV, Pavlicek W. How I do it: managing radiation dose in CT. Radiology 2014;273(3): 657–672

Question 102. Which of the following represents the *best* sequence of events for the "time-out" portion of the Universal Protocol?

A. Time-out is performed before the procedure and initiated by a designated team member. There is active communication among the team with correct identification of the patient and procedure site as well as correct identification of the procedure to be performed. Completion of the time-out is documented.

B. Time-out is performed before the procedure and initiated by a designated team member. Only one individual from the procedure team actively communicates the correct identification of the patient/procedure site and the correct identification of the procedure to be performed. Completion of the time-out is documented.

C. Time-out is performed after the procedure and initiated by a designated team member. There is active communication among the procedure team with correct identification of the patient/procedure site and correct identification of the procedure to be performed. Completion of the time-out is documented.

D. Time-out is performed before the procedure and initiated only by the physician to perform the procedure. There is then active communication among the procedure team with correct identification of the patient/procedure site and correct identification of the procedure to be performed. Completion of the time-out is documented.

Answers:

A—Correct!

B—Incorrect: All members of the procedure team should actively communicate. At a minimum, the team members must agree upon the correct patient identity, the correct procedural site, and the procedure to be done.

C—Incorrect: Time-out is performed before the procedure.

D—Incorrect: Time-out can be initiated by any in the procedure team, including the performing physician.

References

http://www.jointcommission.org/assets/1/18/up_poster.pdf. Published 2016. Accessed March 8, 2016

Lee SL. The extended surgical time-out: does it improve quality and prevent wrong-site surgery? Perm J 2010;14(1):19–23

Angle JF, Nemcek AA Jr, Cohen AM, et al; SIR Standards Division; Joint Commission Universal Protocol for Preventing Wrong Site, Wrong Procedure, Wrong Person Surgery. Quality improvement guidelines for preventing wrong site, wrong procedure, and wrong person errors: application of the joint commission "Universal Protocol for Preventing Wrong Site, Wrong Procedure, Wrong Person Surgery" to the practice of interventional radiology. J Vasc Interv Radiol 2008;19(8):1145–1151

Questions 103 and 104. Regarding perceptual and diagnostic radiological errors:

A. Perceptual error

B. Diagnostic error

Question 103. These are the most common causes of radiological malpractice suits.

Question 104. These are the most common types of radiological errors.

Answers:

103—**B**: Diagnostic errors may be grouped into failures of detection, interpretation, result communication, and appropriate follow-up test suggestions. About 30% of abnormal image findings are missed, although most of these misses are inconsequential.

104—**A**: Perceptual errors are the most common error, accounting for 70% of radiology diagnostic errors. This error occurs when an abnormal image finding is not seen/reported initially but was present in retrospect. Some factors contributing to this error include reader fatigue, rapid reading pace, inconspicuous target lesion, confounding distractions and interruptions, and/or satisfaction of search (search ends inappropriately once one abnormality is found.)

Note: Diagnostic and perceptual errors are interrelated.

References

Donald JJ, Barnard SA. Common patterns in 558 diagnostic radiology errors. J Med Imaging Radiat Oncol 2012;56(2):173–178

Berlin L. Radiologic errors, past, present and future. Diagnosis 2014;1(1):79–84

Questions 105 and 106. Regarding simulation-based training, match the following examples with the type of validity they most closely resemble:

A. Content validity

B. Face validity

C. Predictive validity

D. Construct validity

Question 105. A lumbar puncture technique simulator is used to train first-year radiology residents. Radiologists observe this simulator technique, complete a Likert scale, and agree that it does, in fact, resemble a clinical setting.

Question 106. Medical students and first-year radiology residents (novices) attempt the lumbar puncture technique simulator and are not successful. However, second-year or higher radiology residents (experts) are successful.

Answers:

105—**B**: Face validity. There is similarity between real-life objects and the simulator. In other words, the test appears "valid." A Likert scale is typically used with questionnaires/surveys where the respondent specifies their level of agreement (i.e., strongly agree to strongly disagree) on a scale typically of 1 to 5.

106—**D**: Construct validity. The simulation activity can differentiate operators of varying levels of expertise.

In general, validity involves determining the degree to which a simulation model and its data accurately represent the real-life situations that they are intended to measure. Content validity is when the simulator is able to teach or assess the desired knowledge. Predictive validity demonstrates a correlation between the simulation performance and real-life clinical scenarios. Other types of validity include concurrent and discriminant. Concurrent validity confirms that a particular test does correlate with a previously validated measure. Discriminant validity tests if concepts or measurements that are supposed to be unrelated are, in fact, not related.

References

Gould D. Using simulation for interventional radiology training. Br J Radiol 2010;83(991):546–553

Gould DA. Training on simulators: limitations and relevance. Eur J Vasc Endovasc Surg 2007;33(5):533–535

Rutherford-Hemming T. Determining content validity and reporting a content validity index for simulation scenarios. Nursing Ed Persp 2015;36(6):389–393

Question 107. An organization focuses on building robust communications to protect against unexpected events and errors. This would be described as:

A. A patient safety organization

B. An organization utilizing root cause analysis (RCA)

C. An organizational resiliency effort

D. An organization utilizing benchmarking

Answer:

C—Correct! This is an example of a resiliency effort by an organization. This is a critical system property that allows an organization to bounce back when unexpected events occur. This requires incorporation of methods to potentially detect these unexpected events and a means to adapt and survive. Focus is made on forecasting future events and preparing for them, not focusing on the errors themselves.

The organization must be actively involved in risk management. Factors improving an organization's resiliency include effective communication and input from all stakeholders.

A—Incorrect: Patient safety organizations are involved in reporting the findings of RCAs in aggregate.

B—Incorrect: This is similar to answer choice A.

D—Incorrect: Benchmarking involves measuring quality items of an organization to standard measurements.

References

Leflar JJ, Siegel MH. Organizational resilience. Managing the risks of disruptive events – a practitioner's guide. Boca Raton, FL: CRC Press; 2013

Armour M. Busting myths and building resilience: Practices and approaches that go beyond mere plan development. J Bus Continuity Emerg Plann 2014–2015;8(2):106–113

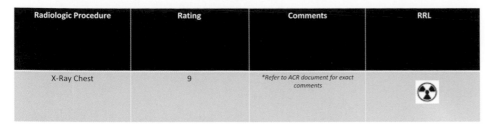

Radiologic Procedure	Rating	Comments	RRL
X-Ray Chest	9	*Refer to ACR document for exact comments	☢

Fig. 2.18 Taken from ACR appropriateness criteria.

Question 108. The following data are taken from the ACR appropriateness criteria (**Fig. 2.18**) and are regarding the radiologic evaluation of acute chest pain and suspected aortic dissection. What does the rating of "9" indicate, and what does the RRL information mean?

A. 9 = Usually appropriate. Relative radiation level is high.

B. 9 = Usually appropriate. Relative radiation level is low.

C. 9 = Usually not appropriate. Relative radiation level is high.

D. 9 = Usually not appropriate. Relative radiation level is low.

Answer:

B—Correct! 9 = Usually appropriate. Relative radiation level is low. The primary purpose of the ACR Appropriateness Criteria is to provide assistance to referring physicians in selecting the appropriate imaging modality given a particular patient's clinical condition. The criteria are evidence based and may also include expert consensus for their development. They are divided into 10 clinical imaging topics with each topic subdivided into clinical variants. Imaging modalities are assigned a rating from 1 to 9 based upon the appropriateness of the modality for the variant under discussion, as follows: 1 to 3—usually not appropriate; 4 to 6—may be appropriate; 7 to 9—usually appropriate. Each imaging modality is also assigned a relative radiation level (RRL) from a 6-point scale (from an adult or pediatric effective dose range) and denoted with a range of no radiation symbol (lowest level radiation) up to five symbols (highest). This example shows just one radiation symbol. All RRLs are based on current literature review as well as input from physicists and radiologists.

Reference

http://www.acr.org/Quality-Safety/Appropriateness-Criteria. Published 2015. Accessed March 8, 2016

Question 109. Which of the following are correct regarding PQRS (Physician Quality Reporting System)? Choose *all* that apply.

A. Participation is voluntary.

B. Prior to 2016, this Medicare system provided cash incentives to physicians who reported quality clinical data for certain predefined measures.

C. Beginning in 2015, negative payment adjustments are now made to the Medicare Physician Fee Schedule if PQRS data for covered services are not satisfactorily reported.

D. PQRS applies to imaging and other specialties.

Answer:

A, B, C, D—Correct! PQRS was developed by CMS as incentive ("bonus") payments to physicians to encourage reporting on specific quality measures. The measures to report on are pre-selected and change from year to year. The incentive amount declines per year. For example, in 2016, a –2% adjustment will be made to the Medicare Physician Fee Schedule for unsatisfactorily reported 2014 data. Participation is voluntary for eligible professionals, whether they participate as an individual physician or as part of a group. PQRS is not intended solely for imaging professionals.

References

https://www.cms.gov/Medicare/Quality-Initiatives-Patient-Assessment-Instruments/PQRS/Downloads/PQRS_Overview FactSheet_2013_08_06.pdf. Published 2013. Accessed March 8, 2016

https://www.cms.gov/eHealth/downloads/eHealthU_PQRSQualityManagement101.pdf. Published 2014. Accessed March 8, 2016

https://www.cms.gov/Medicare/Quality-Initiatives-Patient-Assessment-Instruments/PQRS/index.html. Published 2015. Accessed March 8, 2016

Silva E III. PQRS becoming easier for radiology. J Appl Commun Res 2014;11:442

Question 110. Which is/are true regarding elements of professionalism? Choose *all* that apply.
A. Professionalism is one of the six core competencies of the MOC.
B. Professionalism requires sensitivity to diverse patient populations.
C. Professionalism should measure up to public expectations.
D. Professionalism requires skills obtained via medical school and residency.

Answer:

A, B, C, D—Correct! In addition, professionalism requires skills and competence verified by a certifying board and MOC. It also mandates character which includes preeminence of patient demands (placing the patient's interest at the forefront), a commitment to a global view of healthcare, and an allegiance to appropriately and wisely utilizing healthcare resources. Professionalism requires the physician to seek to improve the quality of healthcare.

References

Madewell JE, Hattery RR, Thomas SR, et al. American Board of Radiology: maintenance of certification. Radiographics 2005;25(1):285–296

Hattery RR, Dunnick NR. Shaping the future: maintenance of board certification and quality care. J Am Coll Radiol 2006;3(11):867–871

Question 111. Which of the following is *not* an element of NPSG's UP.01.02.01—marking a procedure site?
A. Mark the procedure site before performing the procedure.
B. Involve the patient, if possible.
C. Make the mark sufficiently permanent to allow visibility after skin preparation and draping.
D. Use only an adhesive marker when marking a procedure site.

Answer:

D—Correct! An alternative process for marking (besides an adhesive marker) must be available for patients who refuse this or when it is technically or anatomically not possible to mark the site. What the alternative method might be is determined on an institution-by-institution basis.

The remaining answer choices are elements of NPSG's UP.01.02.01. In addition, a licensed independent practitioner who will be present and is responsible for the procedure should mark the site (or a qualified individual delegated by the licensed independent practitioner).

NPSG stands for National Patient Safety Goals, overseen by The Joint Commission (TJC) and established in 2002. The primary objective is improving patient safety. A panel of experts advises TJC on the NPSG, and input is also solicited from practitioners and stakeholders. TJC then prioritizes patient safety issues and tailors the goals (NPSGs) as applicable to a specific accreditation program. There were 16 NPSGs in 2015 which included topics such as identifying patients correctly, using medications correctly, using alarms safely, preventing infection, identifying patient safety risks, and preventing surgical mistakes. There will be no new NPSGs for 2016.

References

http://www.mghpcs.org/RR/Documents/Overview_UP_010201.pdf. Published 2015. Accessed March 8, 2016

Murphy J. Joint commission national patient safety goals. Topics in Patient Saf 2014;14(1):1–2

Questions 112 through 114. In a Just Culture Model, there are three manageable behaviors: human errors, at-risk behavior, and reckless behavior. For each scenario below, select from answer choices A through D on how to best manage these behaviors based upon this model.

A. Console
B. Coach
C. Punish
D. Dismiss

Question 112. A radiologist is under the influence of alcohol while interpreting imaging studies. He calls the ordering physician and reports a life-threatening finding. However, it was actually on a different patient who subsequently dies.

Question 113. A radiology resident follows the appropriate protocol for discussing and obtaining consent with a patient for an IR procedure. He then grabs a marker from a nearby desk and marks the site of the procedure. Before the procedure, the patient sips some ice water, some of which spills on his chest. The patient uses a blanket to wipe the ice water off. The site marked is no longer seen as a nonpermanent marker had been used. In the IR suite, he is sedated before it is discovered that the prior site marking is no longer there.

Question 114. This is the same scenario as in question 113. The physician in charge decides to continue with the procedure anyway, since written notes indicate the correct location.

Answers:
112—**C**: Punish. This is an example of reckless behavior, which is defined as a behavioral choice to consciously disregard an unjustifiable risk. Here, safety norms are willfully ignored. This is managed through punishment—remedial or punitive action.

113—**A**: Console. This is an example of human error, an inadvertent action of doing something other than what should have been done but not intentional. This is a good faith human error rather than negligence. This is managed through consolation via changes in choices, processes, procedures, training, design, or the environment.

114—**B**: Coach. Behavior such as this, where risk is increased but not recognized or mistakenly considered justified, should be coached. This behavior includes "work-around" errors/choices that are made for convenience, but underestimate the risk of the actions taken. Management might include removing incentives for the behavior, creating incentives for better choices, and increasing situational awareness.

A just culture organization identifies the types of behavioral choices that employees make, how the employees should be managed, and how best to hold the employees accountable for the actions. An effort is made to not necessarily place blame on the individual, but at the same time, to hold them accountable for these actions. In the end, this promotes a partnership for patient safety.

References
Boysen PG II. Just culture: a foundation for balanced accountability and patient safety. Ochsner J 2013;13(3):400–406

Abujudah HH, Bruno MA. Quality and Safety in Radiology. New York, NY: Oxford University Press; 2012

Agrawal A. Patient Safety: A Case-Based Comprehensive Guide. New York NY: Springer Science & Business Media; 2013

Question 115. What effect may a steep authority gradient have on an organization's culture of safety?

A. Safety issues may go unreported to upper leadership for fear of retribution punishment.
B. Reported safety issues are more likely to diffuse their way to upper leadership, since there is an excellent chain of communication from lower level to upper level leadership.
C. A steep authority gradient style incorporates a culture of safety at all levels.
D. A steep authority gradient reduces the potential for endangerment of a patient.

Answer:
A—Correct! A steep authority gradient is one where the leader is perceived as a dictator, and team members are not free to question or express concerns. In this type of situation, there is fear of repercussions from reporting safety concerns.

B—Incorrect: The opposite is true. A steep authority gradient results in suboptimal communication.

C—Incorrect: The opposite is true. A steep authority gradient discourages full involvement at all levels for a culture of safety.

D—Incorrect: The opposite is true. A steep authority gradient does not promote shared knowledge and teamwork, and therefore, may endanger patients.

References
Cosby KS, Croskerry P. Profiles in patient safety: authority gradients in medical error. Acad Emerg Med 2004;11(12):1341–1345

Mitchell P, Hampshire MS. Safer Care Human Factors for Healthcare: Trainer's Manual. Argyll and Bute, Ontario: Swan & Horn; 2013

Question 116. Regarding CT imaging and the Image Gently campaign, which of the following are recommended ways to reduce the radiation dose in children? Choose *all* that apply.

A. Scan only when necessary.

B. Scan once.

C. Use last image save mode as often as possible.

D. Scan only the indicated region.

E. Reduce the amount of radiation used.

Answer:

A, B, D, E—Correct! Perform CT imaging only when necessary. Use alternative imaging with less or no ionizing radiation, if possible. Use single phase rather than multiphase imaging. Scan only the body area of interest. Reduce the amount of radiation by "child-sizing" the kVp and mA, adjusting protocols, and comparing equipment doses with the ACR standards (and adjusting, if necessary).

C—Incorrect: This is a technique related to fluoroscopy, not CT. All of the other answer choices are recommended ways of reducing CT radiation dose to children (A, B, D, E).

References

John SD, Moore QT, Herrmann T, et al. The Image Gently pediatric digital radiography safety checklist: tools for improving pediatric radiography. J Am Coll Radiol 2013;10(10):781–788

Don S, Macdougall R, Strauss K, et al. Image gently campaign back to basics initiative: ten steps to help manage radiation dose in pediatric digital radiography. AJR Am J Roentgenol 2013;200(5):W431-436

Question 117. When should medication reconciliation occur? Choose *all* that apply.

A. At discharge

B. At admission

C. At transfer

Answer:

A, B, or C—Correct! Admission, transfer, or discharge—any of the above. Medication reconciliation is a goal (03.06.01) established by the NPSG under TJC. This goal was reaffirmed in 2010 as an important safety issue and should be followed at any point of transition in a patient's care, including admission, transfer, or discharge. This helps to avoid duplication, incorrect dosages, and omission of needed medications.

References

Barnsteiner JH. Medication reconciliation. In: Hughes RG, ed. Patient safety and quality: an Evidence-Based Handbook for Nurses. Rockville, MD: Agency for Healthcare Research and Quality (US); 2008

Daly M, Lee B. Examining medication reconciliation from a perspective of safety. Formulary; 2013;48(8):266–270

Question 118. Patients at higher-than-average risk for an acute allergic-like reaction from intravenous iodinated contrast administration are typically premedicated with a corticosteroid and/or antihistamine. Which are valid reasons to administer the premedication orally at about 4–6 hours before the contrast is given? Choose *all* that apply.

A. It is easier to give oral versus intravenous medications.

B. Reactions from administration of corticosteroids are more likely if given intravenously.

C. There is less evidence of efficacy when given in shorter timeframes.

D. Antihistamine effects begin at about four hours with a maximal effect by eight hours.

Answer:

A, B, C, D—Correct! All of the above. For a patient without contraindication to oral intake and no IV at the time, this is simpler. Maximal effect of oral prednisone begins at 1 to 2 hours after administration, and the half-life is about 4 hours. This fact, along with the best effects from antihistamines being at about 4 to 8 hours (histamine in sedimented leukocytes is reduced by 4 hours with maximal effect by 8 hours), deems giving the premedication at about 4 to 6 hours before contrast injection as an appropriate timeframe (a compromise between the effects of the steroid and the antihistamine). In addition, it is unclear if giving a steroid (oral or IV) at 3 hours or less prior to IV contrast reduces potential adverse effects of the contrast. Greenberger et al reported the risk of repeat anaphylactoid reaction from IV contrast media to be between 17 and 60%.

References

ACR Manual on Contrast Media. V 10.2. 2016. http://www.acr.org/quality-safety/resources/contrast-manual. Accessed September 2, 2016

Greenberger PA, Patterson R, Radin RC. Two pretreatment regimens for high-risk patients receiving radiographic contrast media. J Allergy Clin Immunol 1984;74(4, Pt 1):540–543

CLASS I - NORMAL HEALTHY PATIENT	CLASS IV - SEVERE SYSTEMIC DISEASE THAT IS A CONSTANT THREAT TO LIFE
CLASS II - MILD SYSTEMIC DISEASE	CLASS V - MORIBUND PATIENT NOT EXPECTED TO SURVIVE WITHOUT THE OPERATION
CLASS III - SEVERE SYSTEMIC DISEASE THAT IS NOT INCAPACITATING	CLASS VI - DECLARED TO BE BRAIN-DEAD AND WHOSE ORGANS WILL BE DONATED

Fig. 2.19   Six levels of ASA classification scheme.

Question 119. In general, which ASA (American Society of Anesthesiologists) class patients are qualified for moderate sedation?
A.   II and III
B.   I and II
C.   Only I
D.   III and IV

Answer:
B—Correct! I and II. More advanced disease class patients may require consultation by an anesthesiologist. Non-anesthesiologists are not permitted to perform sedation on Class V patients.

The ASA classification scheme was created in 1963 to help assess preoperative risk in patients based on their overall physical status/ health. It has been found that postoperative complications are closely related to the preassigned ASA class or score. These are the six levels of this classification scheme (**Fig. 2.19**).

References
Daabiss M. American Society of Anaesthesiologists physical status classification. Ind J Anaesth 2011; 55(2):111–115

American Society of Anesthesiologists: https://www.asahq.org/ resources/clinical-information/asa-physical-status-classification-system. Published 2014. Accessed March 8, 2016

Question 120. What is the purpose of a criticality index (as a tool for evaluating risk and adverse events)?
A.   It assists in identifying active errors (critical) versus latent errors (noncritical).
B.   It helps to identify the underlying problems (critical areas) that increase the likelihood of errors.
C.   It gives a rough quantitative estimate of the magnitude of hazard for each step in a high-risk process.
D.   It is assigned to the steps in a high-risk process that must be eliminated.

Answer:
C—Correct! The criticality index is utilized with Failure Mode and Effects Analysis (FMEA) to help the prospective identification of error risk within a particular process. A criticality index is assigned to each step in a process to allow prioritization of targets that need improvement.

A—Incorrect: This answer choice refers to active and latent errors and is not related to the criticality index.

B—Incorrect: This answer choice refers to RCA.

D—Incorrect: The criticality index prioritizes each step in order of need for improvement. The emphasis is on prioritizing, not necessarily eliminating steps.

References
Riplova K. Tool of risk management: failure mode and effects analysis and failure modes, effects and criticality analysis. Journal of Information, Control and Management Systems 2007;5(1):111–120

Petrillo A, Fusco R, Granata V, et al. Risk management in magnetic resonance: failure mode, effects, and criticality analysis. Biomed Res Int 2013; 2013:763186

McElroy LM, Khorzad R, Nannicelli AP, et al. Failure mode and effects analysis: a comparison of two common risk prioritization methods. BMJ Qual Saf 2016;25(5):329–336

Question 121. A teenage girl falls, and there is clinical concern for a left ankle fracture (**Fig. 2.20**). The following study is read as negative. The abnormal soft tissue finding in Kager's fat pad (arrow) is not reported as the interpreter's focus during interpretation was only on a possible fracture. This is an example of which cognitive bias?

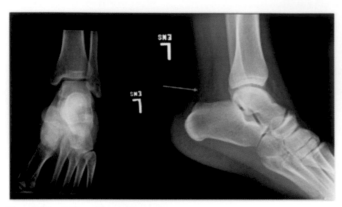

Fig. 2.20 Left ankle radiograph.

A. Multiple alternative
B. Anchoring
C. Search satisfaction
D. Framing effect
E. Premature closure

Answer:

C—Correct! Search satisfaction occurs when one detects an abnormality on imaging, then looks no further, because he/she is satisfied with the search (and, subsequently, misses any additional findings).

A—Incorrect: Multiple alternative bias. This occurs when there is uncertainty of the correct diagnosis because of the multiplicity of differential diagnosis options.

B—Incorrect: Anchoring. This occurs when one is locked into features/findings from an initial presentation for making the diagnosis and fails to adjust the initial diagnosis from information obtained later.

D—Incorrect: Framing effect. This occurs when a correct diagnosis is strongly influenced by how others frame a problem.

E—Incorrect: Premature closure. This occurs when a diagnosis is made before it has been fully verified or thought out.

References

Ha AS, Porrino JA, Chew FS. Radiographic pitfalls in lower extremity trauma. AJR Am J Roentgenol 2014;203(3):492–500

Croskerry P. The importance of cognitive errors in diagnosis and strategies to minimize them. Acad Med 2003;78(8):775–780

Questions 122 to 125. Each of the following reactions occurs after a patient receives IV iodinated contrast. Assuming basic treatment such as oxygen, fluids, monitoring vitals, etc., have already been performed, which is the *best* choice for subsequent medication treatment?

A. Labetalol
B. Atropine
C. Benzodiazepine
D. No medication
E. Epinephrine

Question 122. Anxiety

Question 123. Severe hives

Question 124. Vasovagal reaction

Question 125. Seizure

Answers:

122—**D**: No medication. Look for other causes for anxiety. Otherwise, reassure the patient.

123—**E**: Administer 20 to 50 mg of diphenhydramine IV (slowly over 1-2 minutes) or IM.

124—**B**: Hypotension with bradycardia. If the patient does not respond to elevating the legs, the Trendelenburg position, and/or fluids, atropine can be administered next. The atropine dose is: 0.6 to 1 mg IV slowly; can repeat up to a total dose of 0.04 mg/kg (2–3 mg) in an adult.

125—**D**: The initial step is typically observing and protecting the patient without medication administration. You may need to turn the patient on his or her side to avoid aspiration. If the seizure persists, call the emergency response team and then consider giving 2 to 4 mg of lorazepam (a benzodiazepine) IV slowly, up to 4 mg maximum.

Reference

ACR Manual on Contrast Media. V 10.2. 2016. http://www.acr.org/quality-safety/resources/contrast-manual. Accessed September 2, 2016

Question 126. A High Reliability Organization (HRO) is committed to:

A. Product delivery timeliness

B. A culture of honesty

C. A culture of safety

D. Risk reduction solutions

Answer:

C—**Correct!** Culture of safety. An HRO commits to and attempts to maintain a high level of safety at all levels within the organization. Some elements include a blame-free environment, commitment of resources to address safety concerns, and efforts for all to collaborate in this culture of safety.

References

Edwards MT. An organizational learning framework for patient safety. Am J Med Qual 2016; Epub ahead of print

Larson DB, Kruskal JB, Krecke KN, Donnelly LF. Key concepts of patient safety in radiology. Radiographics 2015;35(6):1677–1693

Ruchlin HS, Dubbs NL, Callahan MA. The role of leadership in instilling a culture of safety: lessons from the literature. J Healthc Manag 2004;49(1):47–58, discussion 58–59

Questions 127 to 131. Regarding the radiologist reading workstation and image retrieval/viewing, match the terms and descriptions.

A. DICOM

B. PACS

C. Luminance

D. Pixel pitch

E. Computer cloud

Question 127. This is a system for image transmission, storage, archiving, review, and manipulation.

Question 128. This is suggested to be 0.20 mm.

Question 129. This is suggested to be at least 350 cd/m² for most diagnostic imaging.

Question 130. This is a means to view images/obtain various services over a network, often the Internet.

Question 131. This is the communications standard for medical imaging.

Answers:

127—**B**: PACS or Picture Archiving and Communications Systems. In addition to the purposes already mentioned, this system allows remote viewing of images (including web-based for teleradiology), integration of quality improvement and performance initiatives, and an interface platform for hospital information systems (HIS), radiology information systems (RIS), and electronic medical records (EMR).

128—**D**: Pixel pitch. This is the physical distance between the pixels on a display and impacts the display resolution and optimal viewing distance. The smaller the pixel pitch, the more pixels are used to display the image. This improves resolution and optimal viewing distance. A pixel pitch of 0.20 means the "dots" are 20/100ths of a millimeter apart. This is the suggested pixel pitch for diagnostic interpretation.

129—**C**: Luminance. This refers to the brightness or the intensity of light emitted per unit area. It is measured in candelas per meter squared (cd/m²). A higher luminance is preferred. For diagnostic monitors, the maximum luminance should be at least 350 to 420 cd/m². Luminance ratio (LR) is the maximum luminance (white pixel) to the minimum luminance (black pixel). Higher LR provides higher contrast. LR should be consistent for all monitors in a single institution.

130—**E**: Computer cloud. This refers to internet-based computing which allows image transmission, storage, servers, and various applications to be utilized by an organization through the Internet. There is a network of servers that are accessed. A cloud is a means of transmitting images from one location to another and serves teleradiology particularly well.

131—**A**: DICOM. This stands for Digital Imaging and Communications in Medicine and is the standard for handling all medical imaging, including data encoding and exchange, storage, transmission, display, archiving, retrieving, etc. DICOM standards are set by the ACR and National Electrical Manufacturers Association (NEMA). Each image file ends with ".dcm"

References

Krupinski EA, Flynn MJ, Hirschorn DS. Displays. ACR IT Reference Guide for the Practicing Radiologist. http://www.acr.org/Advocacy/Informatics/IT-Reference-Guide. Accessed September 4, 2016

Eren H, Webster JG. Telemedicine and Electronic Media. Boca Raton, FL, CRC Press; 2015

Mendelson DS, Rubin DL. Imaging informatics: essential tools for the delivery of imaging services. Acad Radiol 2013;20(10):1195–1212 ftp://medical.nema.org/medical/dicom/2011/09v11dif/09v11_01.doc. Accessed March 13, 2016

Kahn CE Jr, Carrino JA, Flynn MJ, Peck DJ, Horii SC. DICOM and radiology: past, present, and future. J Am Coll Radiol 2007;4(9):652–657

Question 132. Which of the following are *correct* about contrast warming? Choose *all* that apply.
A. It is regulated by the American College of Radiology (ACR).
B. There must be a daily temperature log for each warming device.
C. There must be evidence of regular maintenance of each warming device.
D. Package inserts must include instructions on warming the contrast.

Answer:
B, C, D—Correct! All of these are true about contrast warming. Warmed contrast is easier to inject due to decreased resistance. One article also noted that warmed iodinated contrast reduced the time to reach maximum enhancement duration. Iodinated contrast should be warmed to body temperature (37°C). However, gadolinium-based contrast should be kept at room temperature (15–30°C).

A—Incorrect: Contrast warming is regulated by TJC, not the ACR.

References
ACR Manual on Contrast Media. V 10.2. 2016. http://www.acr.org/quality-safety/resources/contrast-manual. Accessed September 2, 2016

Hazirolan T, Turkbey B, Akpinar E, et al. The impact of warmed intravenous contrast material on the bolus geometry of coronary CT angiography applications. Korean J Radiol 2009;10(2):150–155

Study finds reason to revisit contrast media warming. Health Devices 2012;41(3):94–95

Question 133. The nuclear medicine division of a radiology department measures patient satisfaction for radioiodine treatment at their institution and compares results to the national average. This is an example of:
A. Dashboarding
B. PDSA
C. Benchmarking
D. Value-stream mapping

Answer:
C—Correct! Benchmarking is a technique used when an organization measures a certain performance and compares it to best class companies or other national measures. It is a quality measure for policies, products, strategies, techniques, etc. The purpose of benchmarking is to determine improvement needs, analyze other organizations' successes, and assimilate data to improve performance. As a side note, the ACR has a National Radiology Data Registry to assist with an organization's benchmarking and performance quality measures.

A. Incorrect: Dashboard. This can be related to benchmarking, but a dashboard is the actual physical displaying of the data, not the process.

B. Incorrect: PDSA. This is a four-step internal CQI process and is not necessarily compared to a national standard.

D. Incorrect: Value-stream mapping. This is one of the tools available for lean process improvement and is a visual map of the flow of material and information within a process. This is not a tool for comparing internal quality measurements to national data.

References
Sower VE. Benchmarking in hospitals: more than a scorecard. Quality Progress 2007;40(8):58–60

http://www.acr.org/~/media/ACR/Documents/PDF/QualitySafety/NRDR/NRDRbrochure.pdf. Published 2005. Accessed March 13, 2016

Duszak R Jr, Muroff LR. Measuring and managing radiologist productivity, part 1: clinical metrics and benchmarks. J Am Coll Radiol 2010;7(6):452–458

Question 134. Regarding *p*-values and confidence intervals in scientific studies, which pair of statements is *most* correct?
A. *p*-value: Used to determine whether a value is true or false. Confidence interval: Gives information on the range in which a true value lies with a certain degree of probability, and no information is given on the direction and strength of the effect.
B. *p*-value: Used to determine if a null hypothesis should be modified. Confidence interval: Gives information on the range in which a true value lies with a certain degree of probability as well as the direction and strength of the effect.
C. *p*-value: Used to determine if a null hypothesis should be accepted or rejected. Confidence interval: Gives information on the range in which a true value lies with a certain degree of probability as well as the direction and strength of the effect.

Answer:
C—Correct! The *p*-value is a statistical probability test that measures the evidence against the null hypothesis. (This assumes that any effect seen in the intervention group is due to chance.) A small *p*-value indicates that there is strong evidence against the null hypothesis. The results are statistically significant if the *p*-value is <0.5 (indicating that the result is significant, the null hypothesis should be rejected, and the alternative hypothesis should be accepted). The confidence interval is also statistically derived and is a range of values to include the true value. The typical confidence level selected is 95%, which means that the true value is included in 95 of 100 studies. A narrower confidence interval is more precise. A confidence interval can be used to determine how precise an estimate is. Unlike a *p*-value, the confidence interval also indicates the direction of the effect studied.

References
du Prel JB, Hommel G, Röhrig B, Blettner M. Confidence interval or *p*-value?: part 4 of a series on evaluation of scientific publications. Dtsch Arztebl Int 2009;106(19):335–339

Wang EW, Ghogomu N, Voelker CCJ, et al. A practical guide for understanding confidence intervals and P values. Otolaryngol Head Neck Surg 2009;140(6):794–799

Altman DG, Machin D, Bryant TN, et al. Statistics with Confidence. 2nd ed. New York: John Wiley & Son; 2011

Question 135. Which of the following statements is/are included in the new paradigmatic approach to quality science? Choose *all* that apply.

A. There must be strong support for CQI.

B. The focus is predominantly on physician performance.

C. Professionals are treated as valuable resources.

Answer:

A, C—Correct! in the new paradigmatic approach to quality care. This is also termed "quality in healthcare," where all members of the organization are involved in the continuous effort to meet the expectations of the patients and other customers. This includes three main categories: measuring quality, improving quality, and ensuring that personnel management views employees as valuable resources. Statistical techniques may also be employed in assisting decision-making.

B—Incorrect: Focus primarily on physician performance is the traditional view. The traditional view is too narrow which emphasizes conformance to standards but minimizes how employees and/or physicians can help contribute to meeting organizational goals and the needs of the patient.

References

Shrestha RB. Enterprise imaging: influencing wisely – the path forward for value-based imaging. Appl Radiol 2015

Laffel G, Blumenthal D. The case for using industrial quality management science in healthcare organizations. JAMA 1989;262(20):2869–2873

Harteloh PP, Verheggen FW. Quality assurance in healthcare. From a traditional towards a modern approach. Health Policy 1994;27(3):261–270

Question 136. This question is related to the diagram in **Fig. 2.21**. Which of the following statements is/are correct regarding this methodology? Choose *all* that apply.

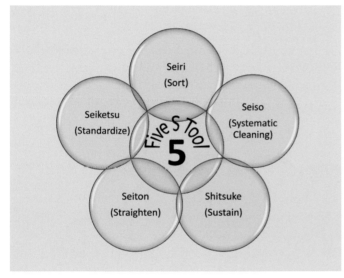

Fig. 2.21 Five S Tool.

A. It was developed in Japan.

B. It is a LEAN management tool.

C. The focus is organizing the workspace with efficiency and effectiveness.

Answer:

A, B, C—Correct! This was developed in post-World War II Japan as a LEAN management tool to organize the workspace, encourage cleanliness, and build a quality work environment. "Five S" stands for a total of five Japanese words that start with the letter "S." Interestingly, they were translated into five English words that also start with the letter "S." Sorting (seiri) means removing unnecessary items and eliminating obstacles. System cleaning (seiso) means "shining" or keeping the workplace clean. Sustaining (shitsuke) means performing regular audits, maintaining discipline, and keeping everything in working order. Straightening (seiton) means to set in order or organize everything into a designated place. Standardizing (seiketsu) means maintaining orderliness and standardizing the best practices (organizational and related to processes).

References

Kruskal JB, Reedy A, Pascal L, Rosen MP, Boiselle PM. Quality initiatives: lean approach to improving performance and efficiency in a radiology department. Radiographics 2012; 32(2):573–587

https://www.creativesafetysupply.com/content/education-research/5S/index.html. Published 2016. Accessed March 17, 2016

Questions 137 to 141. Match the following QI tools with their correct definitions:
A. Walk-through.
B. Brainstorming.
C. Multivoting.
D. Nominal group technique.
E. Prioritization matrix.

Question 137. This is a team exercise that narrows a list of choices to the top priorities.

Question 138. This is when you actually participate in the simulation of processes that the patient encounters.

Question 139. The team ranks the tasks in order of importance.

Question 140. This team tool is used to generate a list of ideas for dealing with controversial issues.

Question 141. This is a team exercise when ideas are openly generated during spontaneous discussions.

Answers:

137—**C**: Multivoting. This is a team decision-making technique when a list of items/tasks is narrowed down by the group to one or more high-priority tasks rather than casting individual votes.

138—**A**: Walk-through. This is a "live" encounter with all the components of a process that a patient would potentially experience such as scheduling the appointment, going to the appointment, arriving at the appointment location, filling out paperwork, sitting in the waiting area, and so on. This can help to identify roadblocks or areas that need improvement.

139—**E**: Prioritization matrix. This is another team tool that sounds similar to multi-voting, but rather than narrowing down the list to one or more high-priority items, the projects are individually given a score ranking them from highest to lowest priority.

140—**D**: Nominal group technique. Every team member has an equal say and vote with little interaction among team members and little influence from domineering members. This technique permits every member of the group to share their ideas and opinions equally. There are two stages: brainstorming and decision-making.

141—**B**: Brainstorming. Brainstorming is not as structured as the other tools listed in this question. It is a freewheeling group discussion used to generate ideas. Unlike nominal group technique, with "brainstorming" there is the potential for domineering personalities to lead the group in their direction.

References

Lipton L, Wellman B. Got Data? Now What?: Creating and Leading Culture of Inquiry. Bloomington, IN: Solution Tree Press; 2012

Shulkin DJ, Otten J. The walk-through patient-focus assessment: preliminary results in augmenting patient satisfaction data. Am J Med Qual 1993;8(2):68–71

Larson DB, Mickelsen LJ. Project management for quality improvement in radiology. AJR Am J Roentgenol 2015;205(5):W470–W477

Boddy C. Nominal group technique: an aid to brainstorming ideas in research. Qual Mark Res 1998;15:6–18

McDaniel JE. Two techniques for alternatives analysis. Radiol Manage 1984;6(2):13–15

Question 142. A breastfeeding mother is to undergo a CTA of the chest to evaluate for possible pulmonary embolism. You are asked to explain and give her data on the safety of doing this study in her situation. Regarding the contrast, which of the statements below can be used to accurately minimize her fears? Choose *all* that apply.
A. Less than 1% of the contrast dose enters breast milk, since contrast agents have poor lipid solubility.
B. The total volume that reaches the infant is <0.01% for iodinated contrast (and incidentally, <0.0004% for MRI contrast agents).
C. There is no radiation in the contrast.

Answer:
A, B, C—Correct! Evidence has shown that such a minuscule amount of contrast enters breast milk and that there is no concern for nursing infants even immediately after the scan is finished. Mutagenic and teratogenic effects have not been described in this clinical situation.

References

ACR Manual on Contrast Media. V 10.2. 2016. http://www.acr.org/quality-safety/resources/contrast-manual. Accessed September 2, 2016

Newman J. Breastfeeding and radiologic procedures. Can Fam Physician 2007;53(4):630–631

Singh N, McLean K. Five things to know about... intravascular contrast media for imaging in breastfeeding women. CMAJ 2012;184(14):E775

Webb JA, Thomsen HS, Morcos SK; Members of Contrast Media Safety Committee of European Society of Urogenital Radiology (ESUR). The use of iodinated and gadolinium contrast media during pregnancy and lactation. Eur Radiol 2005;15(6):1234–1240

Question 143. Regarding a chaperone, which of the following is *not* included in AMA's recommended guideline?

A. A chaperone is only recommended for pediatric and female patients.

B. A chaperone policy should be communicated to the patient, either with a conversation or via a well-displayed written notice.

C. A chaperone must be an authorized health professional when possible.

D. A chaperone must respect patient privacy and confidentiality.

Answer:

A—**Correct!** The AMA guidelines do not specify to which patient populations a chaperone should be made available. A chaperone is an individual who is present during a medical examination or procedure to witness and safeguard both parties, and when possible, should be an authorized health professional. The AMA states that having a chaperone system in place is both ethical and prudent (to provide a secure and safe environment for both the patient and the physician).

References

http://www.ama-assn.org/ama/pub/physician-resources/medical-ethics/code-medical-ethics/opinion821.page. Published 1998. Accessed March 20, 2016

Wong DS. Legal Issues for the Medical Practitioner. Aberdeen: Hong Kong University Press; 2010

Questions 144 through 146 (**Fig. 2.22**). For each term listed, calculate its correct value using the following data.

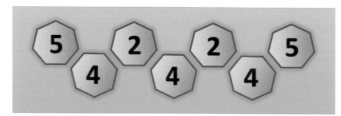

Fig. 2.22   Number listing.

A.   Mean
B.   Median
C.   Mode

Question 144. 3.71

Question 145. 4

Question 146. 4

Answers (see also Fig. 2.23):

144—**A**: Mean. This is also called average. (Sum of observed values)/ (Total number of observations). For this case: (5+4+2+4+2+4+5)/ (7) = ~3.71. This is the best measure of central tendency and is often expressed in literature as *x*.

145—**B**: Median. This is the middle value after all of the observed numbers are arranged from lowest to highest values. This divides the frequency distribution into two halves. It is technically defined as the 50th percentile of the observed values set. For this case, the numbers would be arranged as 2, 2, 4, 4, 4, 5, 5, and the middle or central value is 4. If there is an even number of observed values, then the median is the halfway point between the two middle values. It can be used for determining ratio, interval, and ordinal scale. Median is also not frequently utilized in statistical testing and can be skewed by outliers.

146—**C**: Mode. This is the observed value that occurs the most frequently. There can be more than one mode. This value is not frequently utilized in statistical testing but is the only value that can be used for nominal scale data. It is not generally considered a good indicator of the central tendency. When describing a bimodal distribution, the major mode is the taller peak, and the minor mode is the shorter peak.

These three terms are all measures of central tendency (measurement of the center of the data) and can be used to evaluate sample distribution of the raw data before a full-blown statistical analysis. Determining central tendency is often a good first step in evaluating data, and measuring the data variability is often a good follow-up step. The most important distribution for statistical purposes is the Gaussian normal distribution, which is defined by its mean and SD. The shape of the distribution of observed values determines the position of the measures of central tendency. With a normal distribution, the values are all identical. With a skewed distribution (asymmetric), the mean is at the extreme observation or tail of the distribution, the mode is at the hump of the distribution (indicating the most frequent value), and the median is in between these values (meaning in the "middle"). See the image with examples of a normal distribution and a distribution skewed to the right.

References

Manikandan S. Measures of central tendency: Median and mode. J Pharmacol Pharmacother 2011;2(3):214–215

McCluskey A, Lalkhen AG. Statistics II: central tendency and spread of data. Contin Educ Anaesth Crit Care Pain 2007;7(4):127–130

Sonnad SS. Describing data: statistical and graphical methods. Radiology 2002;225(3):622–628

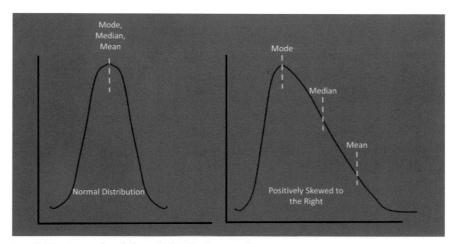

Fig. 2.23   Normal and skewed distribution graphs.

Questions 147 through 149. Match A, B, or C from the image (**Fig. 2.24**) to its best statistical use description.

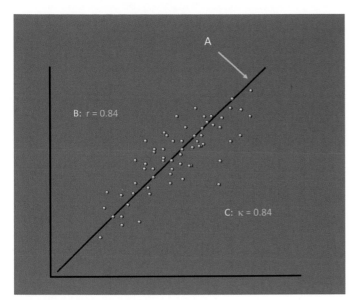

Fig. 2.24 Plotted coordinates on a graph.

Question 147. This estimates the relationship between variables and focuses on a predictor variable of an outcome.

Question 148. This measures the degree of linear association or the strength of the relationship between two continuous variables.

Question 149. This measures the agreement between two or more observers' interpretations and is corrected for chance.

Answers:

147—**A**: Regression line/analysis. This type of analysis mathematically describes the relationship between a continuous dependent (variable Y) and independent variable(s) (variable X). The analysis is made with a scatter plot showing a linear (as in this image) or nonlinear relationship. A straight linear line is defined by this equation: $Y = a + b \times X$, where "a" is the y-intersect and "b" is the slope of the line. The dependent variable can be estimated from the independent variable. Multivariable linear regression analysis can also be performed when the effect of multiple variables on the dependent variable are evaluated.

148—**B**: Correlation coefficient. The correlation coefficient value can range from -1 to +1. The absolute numerical value indicates the magnitude or strength of the correlation. The - or + sign indicates the direction of the relationship (positive indicating direct relationship and negative indicating inverse relationship). The strongest correlation possible is +1. There are two primary types of correlation coefficients: Pearson's and Spearman's. Pearson's is parametric and only used with interval or continuous outcome variables in a normal distribution. Spearman's is nonparametric, used with ordinal or continuous outcomes variables, and is most helpful when extreme values are present, at least one of which is not normally distributed. It describes a monotone relationship when the dependent variable either rises or sinks as the independent variable rises.

149—**C**: Kappa statistic. Ideally, one would desire a k of 1, which would indicate perfect agreement. The closer the value approaches zero, the less agreement there is. Kappa is affected by prevalence. Agreement is not equivalent to accuracy (one can have high agreement but little accuracy). When reading medical literature, keep in mind that the higher the kappa value, the more agreement there is between the interpreters of the test (such as radiological image interpretations), which would make the test more valid and useful clinically.

References

Viera AJ, Garrett JM. Understanding interobserver agreement: the kappa statistic. Fam Med 2005;37(5):360–363

Lang TA, Secic M. How to Report Statistics in Medicine. Philadelphia, PA: ACP Press; 2006

Schneider A, Hommel G, Blettner M. Linear regression analysis: part 14 of a series on evaluation of scientific publications. Dtsch Arztebl Int 2010;107(44):776–782

Yan X. Linear Regression Analysis: Theory and Computing. Singapore: World Scientific; 2009

Questions 150 and 151. Determine which type of bias is represented by each scenario:

A.   Selection bias
B.   Verification bias
C.   Sampling bias
D.   Measurement bias
E.   Confounding bias

Question 150. A retrospective study is performed using previously developed strict inclusion and exclusion criteria. However, due to a smaller-than-expected number of study subjects, the researcher permitted 20 more patients (who did not exactly match the inclusion criteria) to be included.

Question 151. You are studying the incidence of stroke in your hometown. You collect your data by interviewing individuals at a large outdoor rock concert.

Answers:

Bias means that there is a lack of objectivity. Bias influences the outcome or results of a study.

150—**A**: Selection bias. By allowing a few more patients to be included in the study (who did not strictly match the inclusion and exclusion criteria), the patients are now selected in different ways. Randomized controlled studies are less prone to selection bias.

151—**C**: Sampling bias. This is actually a subset of selection bias. You have not likely included several groups in this study. For example, the elderly are either not likely or not able to attend a rock concert. Therefore, you cannot generalize your results to the entire population.

Verification bias (also called work-up bias) occurs when preliminary diagnostic test results affect whether the gold standard test is used to verify these preliminary tests results. Measurement bias occurs when the same measurements are not applied across the board for all patients in a study, and there is measurement error. Confounding bias occurs when the effect of one factor cannot be separated from another factor, thereby making it difficult to demonstrate a causal link between treatment and outcome.

References
Pannucci CJ, Wilkins EG. Identifying and avoiding bias in research. Plast Reconstr Surg 2010;126(2):619–625

Sica GT. Bias in research studies. Radiology 2006;238(3):780–789

Skelly AC, Dettori JR, Brodt ED. Assessing bias: the importance of considering confounding. Evid Based Spine Care J 2012;3(1):9–12

Match the following terms with their *best* description (**questions 152–161**).

A β
B. Type I error
C. Type II error
D. $1 - \beta$
E. Sample size
F. ANOVA
G. *t*-test
H. Null hypothesis
I α
J. McNemar test

Question 152. Compares means from two independent populations (for continuous variables in a normal distribution).

Question 153. Depends on the ratio of the following for the two means being compared: (SD)/(smallest meaningful difference or effect size).

Question 154. The null hypothesis is rejected when it is actually true.

Question 155. The null hypothesis is not rejected when it is false.

Question 156. The probability of avoiding a Type II error.

Question 157. Compares 2+ means from 2+ independent groups.

Question 158. The probability of making a Type II error.

Question 159. What the researcher tries to disprove.

Question 160. The probability of making a Type I error.

Question 161. Compares paired count data.

Answers:

These are some research terms/statistics that you should be familiar with, but not necessarily all the great details.

152—**G**—*t*-test: This is called the paired *t*-test if the same subject is tested at two different times (means from paired samples). There is also the Mann–Whitney *U* test, which compares means from two independent populations for continuous data that are not normally distributed. The Wilcoxon signed rank test compares means from paired samples for continuous data that are not normally distributed.

153—**E**—Sample size: Based upon the ratio given, a decrease in SD or an increase in effect size would decrease the sample size. A predetermined sample size must be made to achieve a desired power level.

154—**B**—Type I error: In other words, the null hypothesis should have been accepted as it is true. This is also called an error of the first kind.

155—**C**—Type II error: In other words, the null hypothesis is accepted, but it is actually false. This is also referred to as an error of the second kind.

156—**D**—1: β or power—If β is the probability of making a Type II error, then $1 - \beta$ is the probability of avoiding a Type II error.

157—**F**—ANOVA (analysis of variance): This is similar to a *t*-test, which compares means from paired samples, but is utilized instead when comparing multiple groups at once.

158—**A**—β: This is the probability of making a Type II error, or failing to reject the null hypothesis when it is false.

159—**H**—Null hypothesis: This is what the researcher tries to disprove, reject, or nullify to demonstrate that there is no relationship (and no statistical significance) between two measured phenomena.

160—**I**—α: For a 95% confidence level, a is typically 0.05 (or a 5% probability) that a true null hypothesis will be rejected (commit a Type I error). As an example, if α is set at 0.02, then there is a 2% chance the null hypothesis will be rejected where it is actually true.

161—**J**—McNemar test: This is for categorical data when comparing paired count data for two measurements from the same subject. The X^2 test is for categorical data for comparison of observed versus expected frequencies. The Fisher exact test is also for categorical data when comparing observed versus expected frequencies, when there is a small sample size of less than 30.

References

Salkind NJ. Statistics for People Who (Think They) Hate Statistics. Thousand Oaks, CA: SAGE Publications; 2013

Elliott AC, Woodward A. Statistical Quick Reference Guidebook. Thousand Oaks, CA: SAGE Publications; 2007

Psoter KJ, Roudsari BS, Dighe MK, et al. Biostatistics primer for the radiologist. AJR Am J Roentgenol 2014;202(4):W365–W375

Question 162. The following mammographic image (**Fig. 2.25**) is an example of computer-aided detection (CAD) where a triangle marks calcifications, and asterisks mark breast masses (*R2 Image Checker*). Regarding CAD in general, which of the following is true?

A. Lowers the rate of false positives.

B. Can substitute for the eye of the radiologist.

C. Can help decrease observational oversights.

D. Utilizes pattern recognition software to identify normal features that are otherwise suspicious to the radiologist's eye.

Answer:

C—Correct! CAD helps decrease observational oversights and improve the detection of suspicious findings (i.e., breast cancer with mammography, lung nodules on CT, etc.). CAD is meant as a supporting role to the radiologist, not a substitute. It helps lower the rate of false negatives. (In fact, CAD marks more false positives than true positives.) CAD utilizes pattern recognition software to identify suspicious features, not normal features, to bring to the radiologist's attention. CAD requires a digital image. Medicare provides additional payment for CAD in conjunction with screening or digital mammography.

References

Castellino RA. Computer aided detection (CAD): an overview. Cancer Imaging 2005;5:17–19

Evolution and Clarification of Computer-Aided Detection (CAD) Coding. http://www.acr.org/Advocacy/Economics-Health-Policy/Billing-Coding/Coding-Source-List/2004/Jan-Feb-2004/Evolution-and-Clarification-of-Computer-Aided-Detection-CAD-Coding. Published 2004. Accessed March 22, 2016

Karellas A, Thomadsen BR. Computer-Aided Detection and Diagnosis in Medical Imaging. Boca Raton, FL: CRC Press; 2015

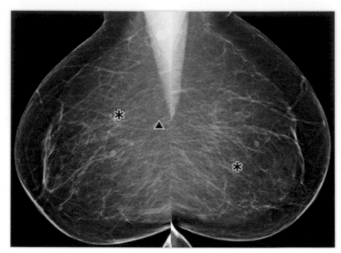

Fig. 2.25　Bilateral MLO mammographic views.

Question 163. The purpose is "to aid the radiology community, individually and collectively, in maintaining a high level of ethical conduct." Where is this statement taken from?

A. ACR Code of Ethics.

B. ACR Principles of Ethics.

C. ACR Rule of Ethics.

Answer:

A—ACR Code of Ethics. This is listed in Article XI of the ACR Bylaws and serves as guidance for physician–patient, physician–public, and physician–colleague ethical and professional conduct. The ACR Principles and Rules of Ethics are subsets of the broader encompassing ACR Code of Ethics. Also outlined are possible disciplinary actions for violations by ACR members, although it is expected that all radiologists follow these guidelines. The principle objective in this code of ethics is to respect human dignity and to do what is in the best interest of the patient.

References

ACR. The ACR 2015–2016 Bylaws. Reston, VA: ACR

Leung AN. Professionalism in radiology. J Thorac Imaging 2014;29(5):284–286, quiz 287–288

Question 164. A young male without risk factors is to undergo a ventilation-perfusion (VQ) scan to evaluate for acute pulmonary embolism (PE). Based upon this limited information, your clinical pretest probability for an acute PE is very low. Which of the following could mathematically assist in determining the pretest probability of this event (acute PE)?

A. Disease frequency ratio.

B. Disease prevalence.

C. Bayes' theorem.

Answer:

C—Correct! Bayes' theorem was originally described by Reverend Thomas Bayes and describes the probability of an event (pretest probability). In other words, the probability of a test result is associated with the absence or presence of a disease (or other relevant information), and this pretest probability can be calculated. In the test population, the pretest probability of disease is the prevalence of the disease.

A—Incorrect: Disease frequency ratio. This would be calculated as: (those who have the disease)/(those who do not have the disease).

B—Incorrect: Disease prevalence. This would be calculated as: [(all new and preexisting cases of a specific disease during a given period of time)/(total population during the same time period)] × 100.

References

Sardanelli F, Di Leo G. Biostatistics for Radiologists: Planning, Performing, and Writing a Radiologic Study. San Donato Milanese, Italy: Springer-Verlag Italia; 2009

Joseph L, Reinhold C. Fundamentals of clinical research for radiologists. Introduction to probability theory and sampling distributions. AJR Am J Roentgenol 2003;180(4):917–923

Question 165. Which is the most effective treatment for contrast extravasation?

A. Elevating the extremity above the level of the heart (to decrease capillary hydrostatic pressure).

B. Apply a warm compress.

C. Apply a cold compress.

D. All of the above.

E. None of the above.

Answer:

E—Correct! None of the above. There is no consensus on the most effective treatment for contrast extravasation. In clinical practice, all of the above treatments (A, B, and/or C) are commonly utilized. It is reported that the incidence of contrast extravasation after power injection for CT is 0.1 to 0.9%. Reported risk factors for contrast extravasation include altered venous access, the inability to communicate adequately, abnormal circulation (including venous or lymphatic), debilitation, or other severe illness. Most cases resolve on their own. Compartment syndrome is the most common complication, and skin ulceration/tissue necrosis is the second most common complication of contrast extravasation. Surgical consultation may be needed in these cases as well as in instances where there is progressive swelling or pain, a change in neurological sensation, altered perfusion, or skin ulceration/blistering.

References

ACR Manual on Contrast Media. V 10.2. 2016. http://www.acr.org/quality-safety/resources/contrast-manual. Accessed September 2, 2016

Tonolini M, Campari A, Bianco R. Extravasation of radiographic contrast media: prevention, diagnosis, and treatment. Curr Probl Diagn Radiol 2012;41(2):52–55

Wang CL, Cohan RH, Ellis JH, Adusumilli S, Dunnick NR. Frequency, management, and outcome of extravasation of nonionic iodinated contrast medium in 69,657 intravenous injections. Radiology 2007;243(1):80–87

Question 166. Dr. Smith is required to undergo a background check prior to practicing medicine at the local university hospital. Which department would this background check fall under?

A. Privileging

B. Criminal background check

C. Credentialing

D. Skills verification

Answer:

C—Correct! Credentialing: This is the application/verification process necessary to gain medical staff admission to an institution, and this occurs before privileging. Some of the items verified or documented include criminal background check, malpractice history, all medical training and board certifications, and peer recommendations. Next, the credentialing application packet is approved by the department chairman, the hospital credentialing committee, and the medical executive committee. The board of directors for the institution grants the staff appointment to the applicant (which is usually a two-year limit, at which time a reappointment application must occur).

A—Incorrect: Privileging. This follows credentialing and involves the applicant requesting specific procedures he or she will be permitted to perform. Documentation to support this is needed. This may include a residency case log, procedure list from a prior institution, or other training documentation. Privileges are also renewed at the time when application is made for reappointment.

C—Incorrect: Criminal background check. This is, in fact, one of the steps included in credentialing.

D—Incorrect: Skills verification. This would be included in the privileging process.

Both of these processes (credentialing and privileging) are required by TJC, with specific details varying by institution.

References

Pelletier SJ, Sheff RA, Cairns C. Core Privileges for Physicians. A Practical Approach to Developing and Implementing Criteria-Based Privileges. 5th ed. Marblehead, MA; HCPro, Inc.; 2010

Eisenberg RL. Radiology and the Law. Malpractice and Other Issues. New York, NY: Springer-Verlag; 2004

Questions 167 through 170. Match the examples given with the type of data/variables they represent.
A. Ratio
B. Nominal
C. Ordinal
D. Interval

Question 167. Age in years.

Question 168. Counts per second.

Question 169. Subspecialty of nuclear medicine.

Question 170. Likert scale.

Answers:

167—**A**: Ratio. This is data on a scale of measurement and can be expressed as a ratio of continuous quantity per unit of magnitude. It is similar to interval data due to an inherent order and uniform size intervals. There is a true zero point, which can indicate the absence of the quantity being measured.

168—**D**: Interval. These data are similar to ratio data as they have an inherent order and uniform size intervals. These data can be averaged and can be continuous or discrete. There is no true zero point.

169—**B**: Nominal. This is the lowest level of measurement, and there is no inherent order to the data. It is simply categorized.

170—**C**: Ordinal. There is inherent order or rank, but no uniform size intervals. The Likert scale is one example where a numerical value is assigned to each choice (ex: 1—strongly agree to 5—strongly disagree).

References

Sullivan GM, Artino AR Jr. Analyzing and interpreting data from Likert-type scales. J Grad Med Educ 2013;5(4):541–542

Marateb HR, Mansourian M, Adibi P, Farina D. Manipulating measurement scales in medical statistical analysis and data mining: A review of methodologies. J Res Med Sci 2014;19(1):47–56

Question 171. An interventional radiologist has been administering Drug A to treat patients with severe procedure-related anxiety. Drug A is not FDA-approved for this use, but rather, only for depression. His well-known procedure is not related to research. He is not aware of any other IR physician utilizing the drug in this manner. He has is now marketing his successful procedure with mention of using this drug in the ads. He fully discloses this to the patients before each procedure and obtains their informed consent. Which piece of information in this scenario is not permissible?

Answer:

This is an example of off-label use of a drug. The FDA prohibits advertising an off-label use of a drug or device to the public. It is acceptable, however, to use Drug A in this manner at his discretion (described in the FDA "practice-of-medicine" doctrine) other than what it was labeled for (whether this be for a different diagnosis, administration route, or patient population). Informed consent is not required except if used in research.

References

Williams J. The first amendment: physician education using off-label indications to ensure that patients receive the most effective treatment. J Med Sci Liaison Society. October 3, 2015. http://themsljournal.com/article/the-first-amendment-physician-education-using-off-label-indications-to-ensure-that-patients-receive-the-most-effective-treatment

Smith JJ. Off-label use of medical devices in radiology: regulatory standards and recent developments. J Am Coll Radiol 2010;7(2):115–119

Question 172. Which of the following was formulated by the Institute of Medicine's (IOM's) Committee on the Quality of Healthcare in America to help achieve/implement the Six Aims for Improvement (STEEEP)?

A. Ten Rules for Redesign
B. Six Rules for Redesign
C. Leapfrog Group
D. None of the above

Answer:

A—Correct! Ten Rules for Redesign. In formulating these rules, the committee "deemed that it would be neither useful nor possible to specify a blueprint for 21st-century healthcare delivery systems." These rules (**Fig. 2.26**) are intended as general principles for redesigning the healthcare system.

References

http://www.nap.edu/read/10027/chapter/1. Published 2001. Accessed March 27, 2016

Kottke TE, Pronk NP, Isham GJ. The simple health system rules that create value. Prev Chronic Dis 2012;9:E49

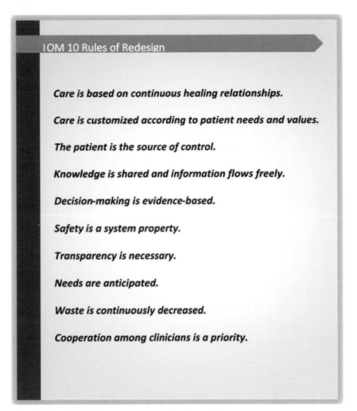

IOM 10 Rules of Redesign

Care is based on continuous healing relationships.

Care is customized according to patient needs and values.

The patient is the source of control.

Knowledge is shared and information flows freely.

Decision-making is evidence-based.

Safety is a system property.

Transparency is necessary.

Needs are anticipated.

Waste is continuously decreased.

Cooperation among clinicians is a priority.

Fig. 2.26 Healthcare system redesign rules.

Question 173. The fundamental principles of the Physician Charter include which the following?

A. Principle of primacy of patient welfare
B. Principle of social justice
C. Principle of free healthcare for all

Answer:

A, B—Correct! The three fundamental principles are A and B above as well as the principle of patient autonomy. These are the common themes by which all physicians should abide and form the basis of their contract with society. The Physician Charter was created jointly by the American Board of Internal Medicine, the American College of Physicians, and the European Federation of Internal Medicine in 2002. Patient welfare: serve the interest of the patient no matter what additional market, societal, or administrative pressures you may experience. Patient autonomy: be honest with and keep your patients informed to enable them to be able to make their own decisions about the healthcare they receive. Social justice: try to eliminate healthcare discrimination and provide healthcare resources fairly to all.

References

Medical Professionalism Project. Medical Professionalism in the New Millennium: A Physicians' Charter. The Medical Professionalism Project from the 2005 RSNA Professionalism Committee. Radiology 2006;238:383–386

Jonsen AR, Braddock CH III, Edwards KA. Professionalism. In: Ethics in Medicine. Seattle, WA: University of Washington School of Medicine; 2014

Question 174. The Chair of your Department of Radiology has created a small committee to oversee implementation of the department's PQRS activities, to include assisting each and every radiologist in the department keep on track in this area. Which physician professional responsibility is he demonstrating by these actions?

A. Commitment to quality of care
B. Commitment to scientific knowledge
C. Commitment to professional responsibilities
D. Commitment to professional competence

Answer:

A—Correct! Commitment to quality of care. There are 10 physician professional responsibilities (or commitments) that follow from the three fundamental principles of the Physician Charter described in the prior question. A commitment to quality of care includes maintaining clinical competence; collaborating with colleagues to reduce medical error, increase patient safety, and improve the outcomes of their care; and minimizing overuse of the healthcare resources. A commitment to scientific knowledge involves upholding and promoting scientific standards and research. A commitment to professional responsibilities entails respecting each other, collaboratively maximizing patient care, and participating in the process of self-regulation to include remediation and discipline of your colleagues who do not meet the professional standards. Commitment to professional competence requires one to commit to lifelong learning and obtaining and maintaining the medical knowledge and skills to, remain competent in your field. The other commitments are maintaining trust by managing conflicts of interest, just distribution of finite resources, improving access to care, patient confidentiality, maintaining appropriate relations with patients, and honesty with patients.

References

Medical Professionalism Project. Medical Professionalism in the New Millennium: A Physicians' Charter. The Medical Professionalism Project from the 2005 RSNA Professionalism Committee. Radiology 2006;238:383–386

Jonsen AR, Braddock CH III, Edwards KA. Professionalism. *Ethics in Medicine*. University of Washington School of Medicine; 2014

Question 175. An Institutional Review Board (IRB) is a formally designated group to review and monitor research related to human subjects. As such, which of the following are the requirements for an IRB? Choose *all* that apply.

A. Approve, disapprove, or require modifications to research.
B. Ensure steps are in place to protect the rights and welfare of the human subjects in the research.
C. Register with the Department of Health and Human Services (HHS).
D. Have a diversity of IRB members.

Answer:

A, B, C, D—Correct! Typically, each institution will have its own IRB. If not, the FDA allows an outside IRB to fulfill this role. An investigator may also be a member of its own IRB, but that investigator cannot participate in review of his or her own protocols/research projects.

References

Labaree RV. Working successfully with your institutional review board. College & Research Libraries News 2010;71(4):190–193

http://www.fda.gov/regulatoryinformation/guidances/ucm126420.htm. Published 2016. Accessed March 27, 2016